Walking on Wheels

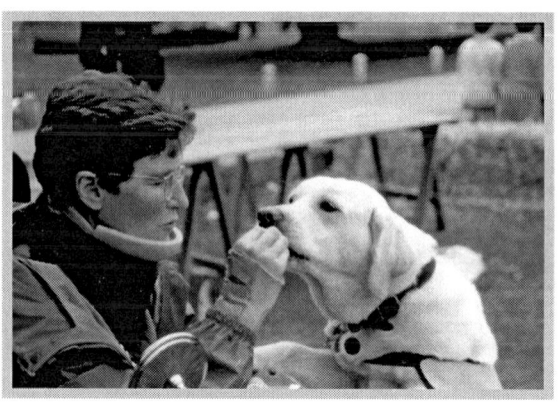

Jill Brown

First published in the United Kingdom in 2011
by The Hobnob Press, PO Box 1838, East Knoyle, Salisbury, SP3 6FA
www.hobnobpress.co.uk

© Jill Brown, 2011

The Author hereby asserts her moral rights to be identified as the Author of the Work.

All rights reserved. No part of this publication may be reproduced, stored in a retrieval system, or transmitted in any form or by any means, electronic, mechanical, photocopying, recording or otherwise, without the prior permission of the publisher and copyright holder.

British Library Cataloguing in Publication Data
A catalogue record for this book is available from the British Library

ISBN 978-1-906978-25-9
Typeset in Minion Pro 12/16pt. Typesetting and origination by John Chandler
Printed by Lightning Source

Contents

Acknowledgements and Dedication   v

1. The Birthday Mouse ~ Early Childhood Memories and Teenage Years   1
2. Office Junior in London   26
3. To King's   31
4. Working towards Qualification ~ 1961   38
5. My Final Year   52
6. To Work in Liverpool   60
7. To Alder Hey and the Best of My Working Days as a Physiotherapist ~ 1965-68   77
8. The Rot Sets In ~ 1968-69   100
9. To Birmingham   111
10. My Career in the Balance ~ 1971-74   126
11. Confusion ~ May 1974 – June 1976   142
12. Problem Solved ~ Diagnosis July – December 1976   153

Epilogue ~ The Way Forward   162
Index   186

Acknowledgements and Dedication

My thanks to Dr. Alex Paton, a good friend who helped me at a very difficult time and later encouraged me to write this book, and edited it for me.

This book is dedicated to my parents, family and friends, including those with four legs, who have all encouraged me to keep walking even when times are difficult.

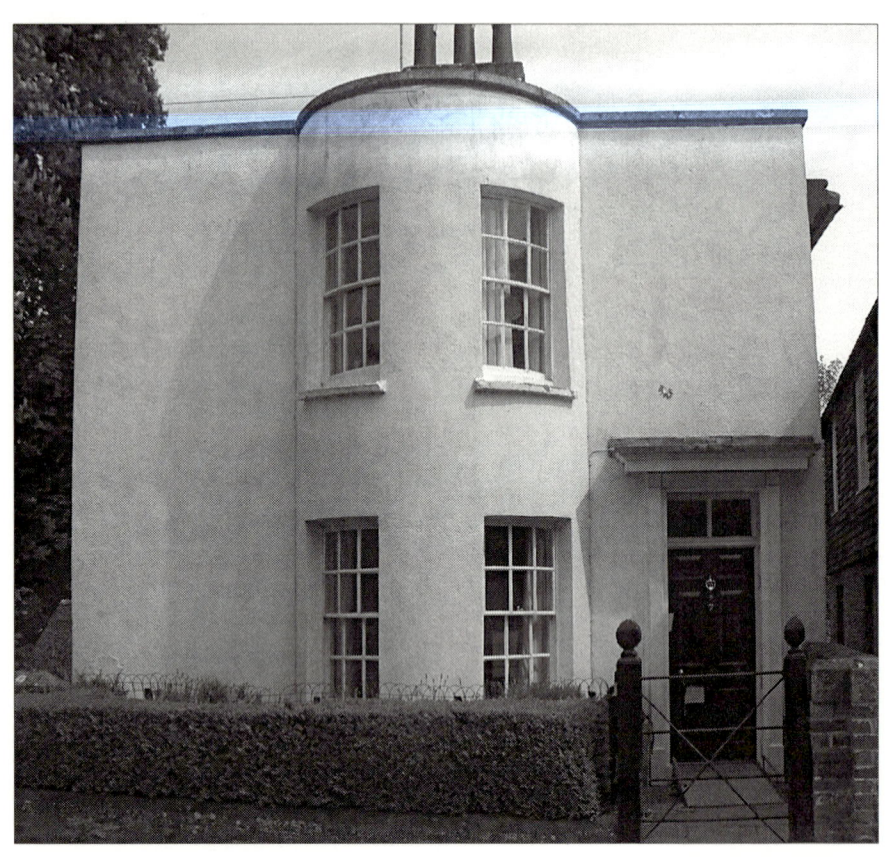

The former St John's Chapel on Harnham Bridge, Salisbury, the home of Jill Brown since 1977

1
The Birthday Mouse ~ Early Childhood Memories and Teenage Years

I HAD A VERY happy and healthy childhood, though I can't remember much of my life before I was five years old when we moved to Blackheath, south-east London in 1946. My father had been appointed Assistant Secretary to the South London Church Fund and we had a most attractive, detached, Queen Anne style house, which 'went with the job', in Kidbrooke Grove. I had been born in the vicarage of St Michael's Church, Ludwick Way, Welwyn Garden City, Hertfordshire on 22nd May, 1941.

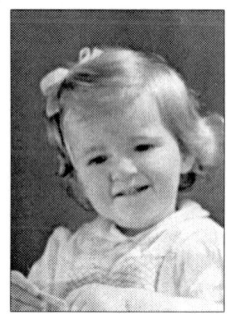

Polyphoto of Jill

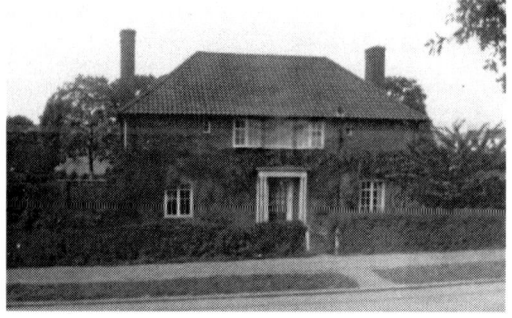

The Vicarage, Welwyn Garden City, my birthplace

It was my eldest sister, Elisabeth's, fifth birthday and apparently when she heard my first cries in the early hours of the morning she thought she had a mouse for her birthday. When I was six weeks old I caused my parents great anxiety having caught whooping cough from my older sisters, but apart from that I was a healthy baby. When friends ask, 'Where on earth is Welwyn Garden City?' I tell them it was the home of Shredded Wheat, which satisfies curiosity immediately. Most of what I know of my early years is from subsequent visits to Welwyn with my parents, who were always welcomed back with great affection. We still have friends from those years and from Luton where my parents grew up and were married, and since my parents' deaths I have continued to correspond with some of them, who have known me since I was a 'bump'.

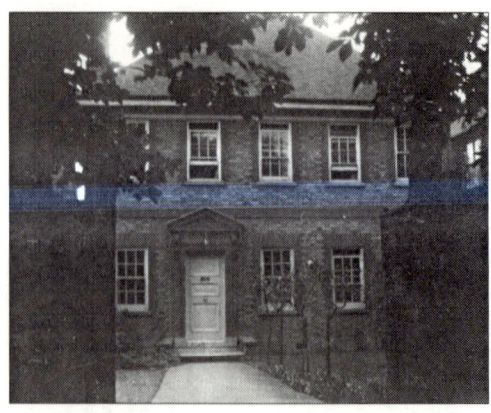

31 Kidbrooke Grove, our London home

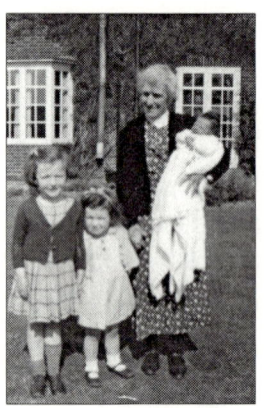

Jill in Granny Brown's arms with her sisters Elisabeth and Petrena

As my hair was almost white I was known as 'Blondie' to parishioners but when we arrived in London I was gradually getting darker and became 'Jill'.

Petrena, my older sister's name, is unusual and rare. My parents were hoping for a boy and as the baby's expected date of birth was June 29th, St Peter's Day, he was to be Peter. However 'Peter' was another girl and she arrived a day early. The curate immediately decided to do some research, and was delighted to find the name 'Petrena'

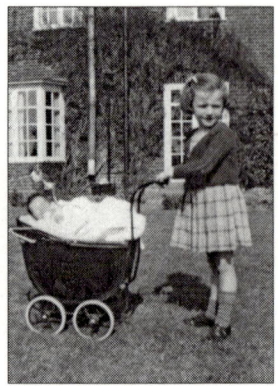

Elisabeth, aged 5, pushing Jill in her doll's pram

- 2 -

which my parents agreed was perfect. When I was born my parents were determined to choose a name which couldn't be abbreviated, as my older sisters names were reduced to Lis and Trena. So Jill it was though when Elisabeth was a teenager she called me 'Jay'.

We have always had a family dog, hence my happiness with them, and there are many photos in the family albums of me with the current dog. I remember sitting in the cupboard under the stairs in Welwyn with our spaniel, Ben, during thunderstorms and air raids, as the vicarage was quite near De Havilland's aircraft company. I don't remember any fear – just the comfort of cuddling my soft, warm companion. When we moved to Blackheath the habit continued, and since adulthood night storms have caused me to huddle under the bedclothes.

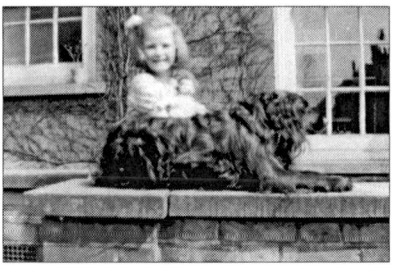
Jill with Ben on the verandah at our home

As Assistant Secretary of the South London Church Fund (SLCF) Father had a 9–5 job in theory and an office in Whitehall. The latter was a wonderful viewing point for royal processions including the Coronation, and we made good use of it. Father's job was a great contrast to his former work as a parish priest, but he soon became involved with All Saints, Blackheath and helped Canon Green with services when he could. His SLCF work involved visiting war-damaged churches in the Southwark diocese to assess the state of church and parish and to discuss with the vicar future plans for any rebuilding and development. He also made site visits with the diocesan architect, then drew up reports and assessments for his boss, Archdeacon Anderson, who was a friendly person and known to us as Andy (so we named one of our dogs after him). Eventually they made decisions about which churches would be repaired and which made redundant. Father also went to churches throughout the diocese to preach about his work and appeal for

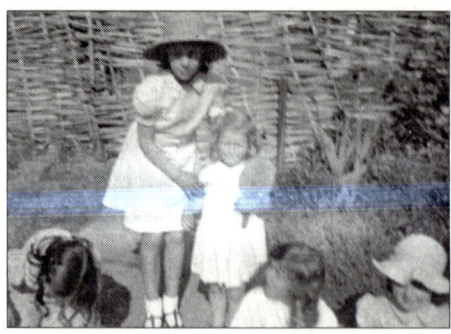
Jill by the garden pond, holding hands with an older parishioner

funds for repairs.

My sisters and I attended St. James Church, Kidbrooke, and joined the Brownies and Guides at appropriate ages. My first school was Blackheath and Kidbrooke School where I went at the age of six; Petrena and I walked to school and collected her friend, Barbara, en route. Blackheath was a pleasant suburb at that time, and although we had main roads to cross – the A2 amongst others – traffic was much less and there was never any question of our being accompanied. Once we were caught in a thunderstorm on our way home and we were so frightened that we knocked on the front door of the nearest house and were given shelter. Oh, that children were safe to do that nowadays.

We were a close family. On Saturdays while Elisabeth and Petrena were busy with Mother I helped Father maintain our very old Austin 7 car – NJ 506 – affectionately known as 'No Joke'. He never was a handy man, let alone a mechanic, and when he became frustrated with his lack of skill it was best to leave him. Another Saturday occupation, in summer, was a visit to Charlton open air Lido where Father tried to teach me to swim. We went on his bicycle and I perched on the cross bar until I had my own bike. Unfortunately I was not a natural swimmer and any progress was rapidly dashed by a thoughtless young lad who ducked me under water when Father wasn't watching. Eventually I had to learn to swim adequately for my First Class test at Girl Guides; I always preferred land sports.

Some Saturdays I went with Father to visit the bombed churches in South London. This could have been boring or depressing but I enjoyed climbing among the brickwork and up scaffolding with him and the architect. My interest in architecture stems from those days when I was taught the rudiments of styles. We went to Southwark

Cathedral on Saturday afternoons for choral evensong since Father had been promoted a Residential Canon and one of his duties was to be responsible, or 'in residence', for all services during his elected months. To make the journey more interesting I collected the names of the public houses along the Old Kent Road in my 'Pub' notebook; it made fascinating reading when I re-discovered it some time after.

We took Mother's home-made scones for the visiting clergymen whom we entertained in the Chapter rooms and someone had to slip out of the service before the end to put on the kettle for tea. My love of cathedrals and church music started at that time, and I still have great affection for Southwark Cathedral, nestling among the Borough Market and railway lines to Waterloo and Cannon Street. We were allocated seats when the Maundy Thursday service was held there, and as the youngest of the family I sat proudly on the nave end of the row, where HRH Prince Philip's shoulders brushed my side. Father, together with other recipients, was presented with a set of Maundy money, which we shared and I still have mine. (He was invited to celebrate the 50th anniversary of his priesthood at Southwark Cathedral in the 1980s. We parked our cars in Borough Market, much altered from my childhood days when we bought fruit cheaply from the 'barrow boys'.) Occasionally we had tea at Lyons Corner House opposite the Cathedral, which was a treat as we rarely had meals out.

Bertram Simpson was Bishop of Southwark when Father was appointed to London. He was a very gentle person and in our family was known as 'Bertie'; I was confirmed by him when I was a teenager. He preached about 'The Good Shepherd' and that was a reflection of Bertie himself, for he was a truly pastoral bishop. His daughter, Joan, looked after him and we kept in touch for many years after his death. When Archdeacon Anderson moved on, Father was promoted to secretary, and Canon Houghton – Reggie – became his assistant. He was sandy haired and very small, probably no taller than five feet, but he had a great sense of humour and often told us jokes.

Shopping was a favourite occupation in those days. Our nearest shops were in Delacourt Road, but the most interesting were in Blackheath village which meant a bike ride across the Heath. I regularly went to the Co-op shop for groceries, handing in ration books although this was post-war Britain, and getting the 'divi' stamps which could be exchanged for goods at the end of the year. There was a wonderful sweet shop near the Co-op where I spent my pocket money on sherbet lemons – what a lovely refreshing fizz when you got to the centre – or a sherbet fountain which had a liquorice tube to suck up the sherbet. When I went back to Blackheath after some years I was amazed to see how much it had grown and how 'up market' the shops had become, but it still retained the village atmosphere.

I also helped mother, who was not very well in those years, with housework which included scrubbing the red kitchen tiles, a satisfying task; afterwards she would apply cardinal red polish. Petrena and I happily shared our large bedroom, which we had to keep tidy. That wasn't hard for me as I have always been a fairly orderly person. Our maternal grandfather, William Marshall, came to stay from time to time. He worked in one of the hat factories for which Luton was renowned. Since the early death of his wife, his unmarried sisters, Lizzie and Becky, who were very upright with their hair in 'buns', went to live with him. They kept house for him and my mother, an only child after the death of her brother from peritonitis when he was twelve. Grandpa was a great smoker and he used to sit by our kitchen boiler rolling his own cigarettes. He was very strict about our shoes: as well as buying us Clark's or Startrite for birthdays and Christmas, he made sure we

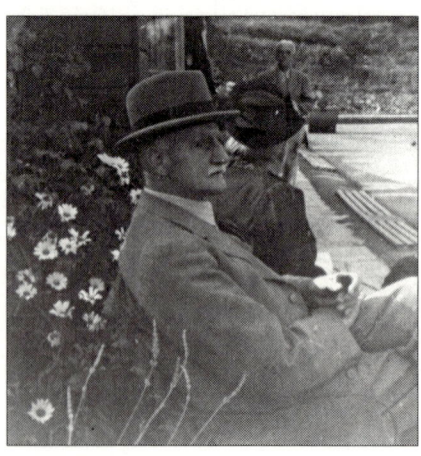

Grandpa Marshall, my Mother's father

cleaned them each day before school. I have him to thank for my lifelong habit of making sure my shoes are clean before going out and of buying decent shoes whatever the cost. At least I still have straight toes.

Lying in bed on hot summer evenings when it was too hot to be covered even with a sheet, we listened to our parents chatting on the verandah beneath our window.

Another familiar noise from our Blackheath days was that of one of our neighbours, Auntie Millie, who lived with her sister-in-law Mrs McPhail, calling her very fat cat in at night. The cat was named 'Poppy poo pah' and to this day I can bring to mind the call, 'pop pop pop poppy, poppy poo pah, poppy poo pah' floating in the air. When Poppy was very slow the calls became frantic and we knew that the cat would be in trouble. I used to visit Mrs McPhail of whom I was very fond, and I was teased over a conversation about handkerchiefs, which she had repeated to my parents. Apparently I told her that I would blow my nose night and morning only, unless I had a cold, so I didn't need many clean handkerchiefs; she used to have lovely, white, lace ones. On one of my visits I was offered a piece of crystallised ginger which defeated me: I had taken the largest piece and put it in my mouth, and the horror of the hot taste meant that I could never subsequently face anything tasting of ginger.

We were fortunate to have good neighbours in Blackheath and I am still in touch with Peter Pichler, who was born during the early 1950s. His parents were hoteliers in London which kept them very busy, and Mary, the eldest child, and then Peter used to envy my parents, who were always at or around our home. As Mrs Pichler went to help in the hotels, the children had a succession of nannies: many were foreign and rather large. Peter used to wait for me to come home from school to play with him, and sometimes there were exotic gateaux from the hotel which we were invited to share. As Father's income was very modest we never had such luxuries at home. Mrs Pichler also gave regular parties and we were invited to share the spread of rich food, as well as to accept any leftovers. Peter adored my parents and used to sit on his rocking horse which he rocked violently, smoking his clay pipe like Uncle Brown, as he called Father, who was a pipe smoker. Mr Pichler gave piano recitals to his friends from London which we had to listen to. At Christmas and birthdays he bought me a new dress and I

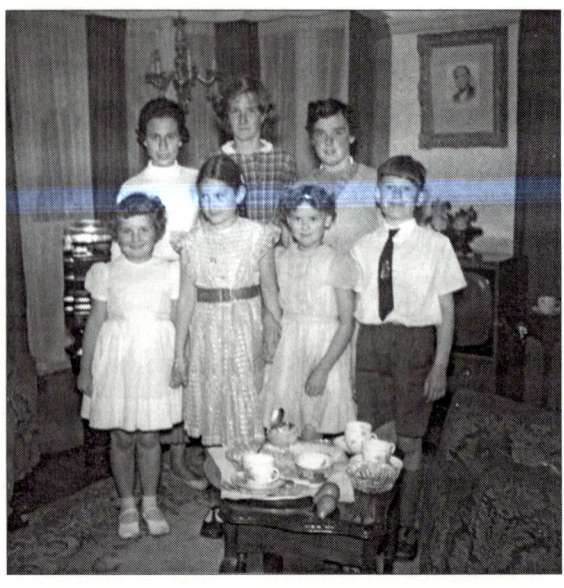

The Pichlers party- Jill, the tallest, in the centre of the back row with Mary in front of her and Peter on the far right of the group

had to go to Daniel Neal in London to make my choice. As I was the youngest in our family most of my clothes were 'hand-downs', so a new dress was really special.

Christmas in Blackheath and Boxing Day tea parties at either our home or at our nearby friends, the Henkels, are happy memories. Mr Henkel was a Lay Reader at All Saints Church, and a baker, and Mrs Henkel a good cook so we always had lovely cakes and buns. Their daughter, Mary, was a year younger than Elisabeth and in the parallel form to Petrena; she was extremely clever and good at both academic studies and sports. She subsequently went to Cambridge where she obtained an outstanding degree in classics. The Henkel's son, Martin was a little younger than me.

On Boxing Day the men went to watch the rugger match between Blackheath and France, while the rest of us played games. A family favourite was 'How green you are'. The rules for this are that one person is elected to leave the room, then the others, the team, choose an item which the elected person must identify. When the team start singing the words 'how green you are' to an easy tune the elected person returns, and is guided to the chosen item by the decibels of the singing. When near the item, the singing is louder and if the person goes away the singing gets softer. The reward for locating the item is the privilege of choosing the next person to leave the room. Another favourite, which suited our home, was 'balloons'. Our hall was a sizeable rectangular room with a curved sweeping stairway up to a small landing which overlooked the hall. We had two teams: those downstairs had to prevent the team on the stairs and landing from bouncing the balloons on to the hall floor.

Our family were all keen cyclists and I had my sisters' hand-down bicycles, until I decided to save my pocket money for one of my own. I still have that 'adult bike' which I bought second hand for ten shillings and sixpence(£0 52½); a few years ago when it wasn't safe for me to ride on roads, I cycled around the local park for short, flat, exercise outings. When I had to give up, Father, by then retired, used it to get to Salisbury Cathedral and the shops. I then had a 'static bicycle' to exercise my legs, but alas, that is no longer possible. When I was 11 or 12 and safe on my bicycle, Elisabeth and I rode off to the country, for example, along the Sidcup bypass to Chislehurst where we had our picnic tea on the Common.

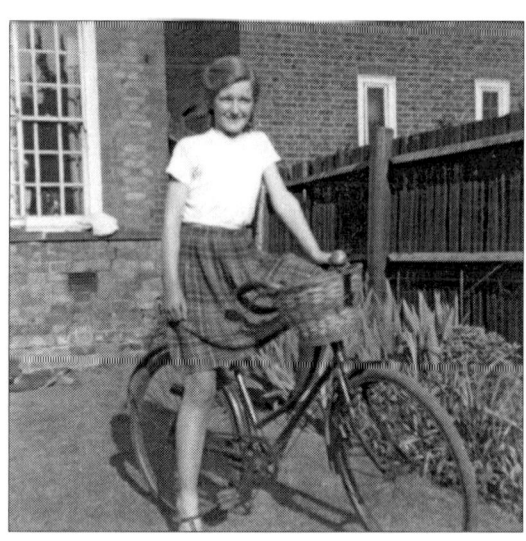

Jill on her bicycle

School Days

Petrena was always a loner and more studious, and apart from walks to school and playing piano duets, I don't recall many activities together. We both had piano lessons, after I got my free place at the High School, with a Miss Morton, quite a large lady, who patiently put us through our paces of scales and pieces at her home. Sometimes we had lessons at school, and I was able to escape art classes, which I didn't much enjoy as I was never an artist. The opportunity of learning the piano gave me a lasting love of music, both to listen to and to play. When I was about 10 we had to write an essay about 'What we would like to do when we grow up' and I am now amused to find that I wanted to conduct an orchestra, though even when I later played in amateur orchestras I never had that ambition.

When I was eight Petrena was awarded a free place at Blackheath High School. As my parents didn't feel happy for me to walk to school alone, they sent me to the fee-paying junior house of the High School

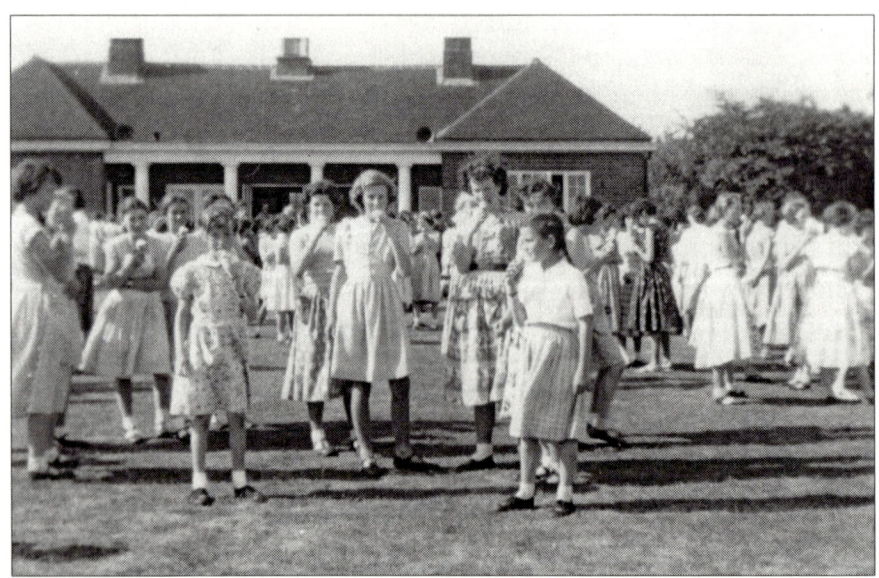

Jill –centre- enjoying an ice cream at the school party

in a large old house near home, so I was allowed to walk or cycle there and back for lunch on my own. I was happy at school and had plenty of friends; the teachers were kind and Miss Lane in particular, who was the form teacher and taught us all subjects apart from Art, made

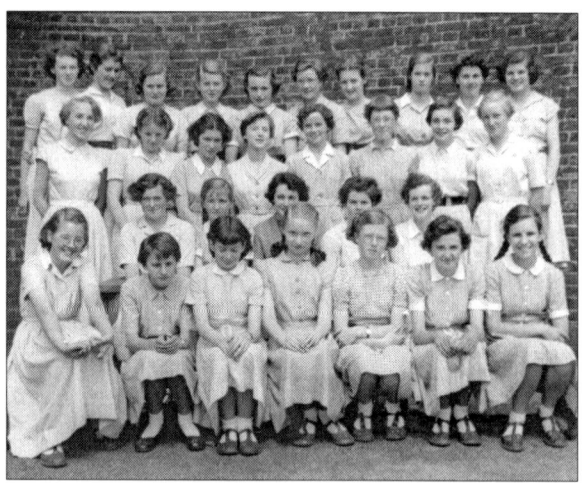

Blackheath High School class photograph 1955. Jill is on the right of the teacher

a great impact on me by her calm manner. The school had a large garden with many bushes and during the summer we spent a lot of time out of doors. At the age of ten I went to the main school in Wemyss Road near Blackheath village, and cycled to school across the Heath from then on. Our school uniform included a Panama hat in summer and velour one in winter, anchored by elastic under the chin; I really disliked the hats and usually pushed them behind my neck but if a prefect was seen, I had to pull the hat quickly into position; wearing a hat incorrectly was a punishable offence which a prefect would report to the Headmistress who would reprimand the offender.

In cold weather the pond on the Heath froze over, and we enjoyed sliding on the ice. My friend Gillian, whom I met at school, had skates but I was happy to make do with sliding in my shoes. In the years of my schooldays between 1947 and 1959, dense smogs frequently covered the Heath. On one occasion we couldn't see in front of the car; to our horror we found that Father was driving across the heath itself (we had thought it was rather bumpy).

In 1952, when I was eleven I too was awarded a free place at the High School, as Petrena had been, and continued there until 17 when I left with 9 'GCE' passes, including additional mathematics. Evening classes in physics and chemistry followed at Woolwich Polytechnic. At school I worked hard and enjoyed lessons, especially mathematics at which I excelled, and Latin. I regularly gained over 90% in mathematics examinations and once 100%. I was in the school choir and sang in the Christmas carol concert each year. In the senior choir we dressed in black cloaks, carried lanterns and processed to the Hall, which was in darkness; there we stood on the stone staircase singing carols. The school had a tradition of making and playing bamboo pipes; I lent mine to a teacher friend in Crosby, Liverpool and never had it back.

I was good at sport and played in the netball and tennis teams for most of my school career. As I was tall for my age I was regularly put as goal defence at netball. I hated lacrosse as my hands were always cold (as they are now), so did Gillian, and as soon as we were able to give up we joined the Priory Squash Club in Blackheath Park and started playing there. I continued in Liverpool (after we moved in 1960 when Father was appointed Bishop of Warrington) until my arm problems became too severe, even playing ambidextrously. I had a good reach and delighted in making my opponents run round me, a tactic which stood me in good stead and got me up the 'squash ladders' in both clubs. I treasure a china mug, which I won at the Northern Club in Crosby for winning the Plate. It doesn't seem possible now, when I can't lift my arms at all nor walk unaided, that I was able to rush round a squash court. I also enjoyed tennis and was given coaching at Wimbledon Park in the Easter holidays: my claim to tennis fame. I was reserve for the first team at school and had a place in the second for a couple of years. In our first house in Liverpool we had a court in the garden which was very convenient, and I continued playing until illness prevented me. I never liked gym; I think my illness must have been lurking at that time for I always found difficulty in climbing ropes and supporting myself on my arms, and tried to avoid those activities from an early age.

Another activity which I much enjoyed was the Girl Guide Movement. As Father had been involved with the Scouts since his childhood, Brownies and then Guides were a natural part of my life and I was an enthusiastic member. In Guides I went from being one of the patrol

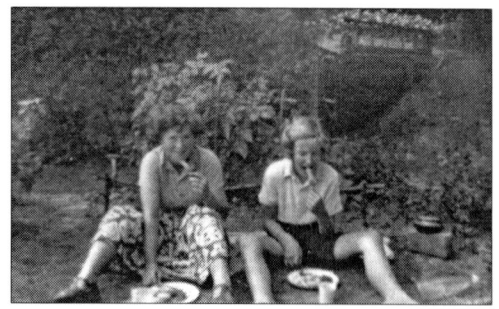

Jill with Gillian eating campfire-cooked sausages in the garden

to a Second, then Patrol leader, and carrying with pride the Colours at Church Parade. My arm was soon covered in proficiency badges and my friends and I revelled in the challenges. I didn't want to camp but enjoyed the day visits to see my sisters when they were camping, and also visits with Father to scout camps. When we visited Elisabeth we had to take a home made bread pudding; Father requested a tin of baked condensed milk (Mother put the tin of condensed milk in a warm oven for about an hour which made the milk more 'gluey').

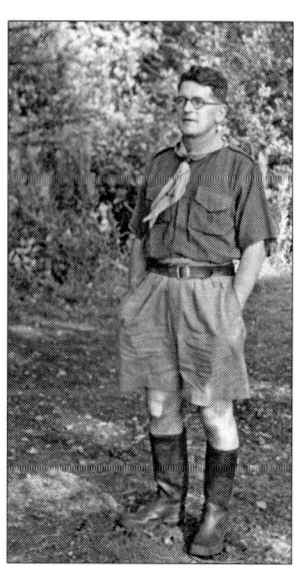

My Father in his Boy Scout uniform

As a Junior Guide I went with my Patrol leader on her ten mile walk; she chose an unusual route from Blackheath to the Tower of London, where we had our photographs taken with a Beefeater. Father became Chaplain to the Scout Movement in London, and I went with him to camps at Westerham, Kent, and Gilwell Park in Epping Forest, Essex. Services in the open air seemed so right, to be thanking the Lord for creation and our lives, with the birds singing around us and the fresh smell of the woods.

Father was asked to christen two of ornithologist Peter Scott's children on board 'Discovery', which was at that time used by the Scouts and moored in London on the Thames. He used the upturned ship's bell as the font and after the service was asked what his fee was. Father said 'nothing', but when pressed said he would like a postcard with a drawing by Peter Scott. A few months later a most beautiful picture of ducks taking off in flight arrived, which I treasure to this day. On another occasion our family was invited to Windsor Castle where Father was presented by the Queen with the Silver Fox, in recognition of his services to scouting.

As a family we usually went for a Sunday afternoon walk with our dog, and living near Blackheath and Greenwich Park we had plenty of choice. I particularly enjoyed the walk to Greenwich and the waterfront at the Naval College; the view from General Wolfe's statue in the Park, near the 24-hour clock and Greenwich Meridian, still holds a fascination for me, though it has changed greatly.

Canine Friends

WHEN OUR FIRST dog, Ben, died, we were all very upset and decided we couldn't have another. However, three months later we acquired a flea-ridden puppy who we called Andy. I was about 10 and we were on a family holiday at Hungtingfield, Suffolk where Father was doing a locum. He had gone to meet our friends the Wilsons, outside Heveningham Hall (I won't forget that unusual name in a hurry). Susan Wilson was my sister Elisabeth's best friend at school and her family were staying at nearby Southwold. When Father returned he confessed that he had brought back a tiny, black and tan, mongrel puppy. While waiting at the bus stop, a young lad passed by on a bike, and

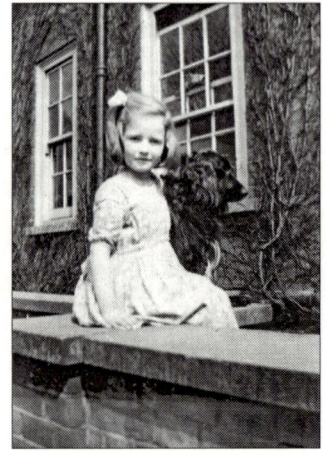

Jill With Ben on the verandah

✳ *The Birthday Mouse* ✳

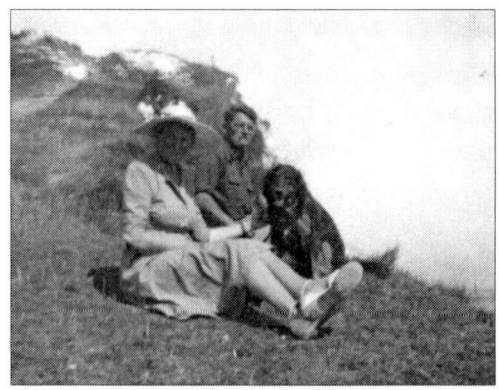

My parents with Andy on holiday

Father asked him if he knew when the bus was due. He noticed a little black head peeping from a cardboard box on the lad's handlebars, and the lad told him his father had sent him to market to buy a puppy, but he had been forced to buy two and the second would be destroyed when he got home. That was enough for Father, so Andy became a much-loved member of our household for the rest of his 14 years. His one fault was that he didn't like car journeys and would put his head out of the window and bark. Andy was our faithful companion until shortly before we moved to Liverpool, and when I returned home for a holiday (I was living in London at the time, completing my physiotherapy training), Judy was in residence – a snappy little Welsh corgi, who was independent and aggressive. She would hang on to Father's cassocks when he went up and down stairs at our Sandfield Park home in Liverpool; in Crosby she was no more agreeable, keeping constantly on the alert for Albert, the cat we'd acquired when we took over the house. She had one place of truce with Albert: in my aunt's room where the two animals would lie together in front of the electric fire. She survived Liverpool and the move to Birmingham, but was getting old and

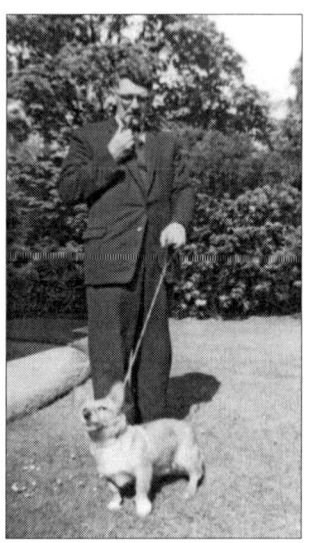

My Father with Judy

crotchety, and often snapped at members of the family, and had to be put down when she developed heart problems.

Three months elapsed when we vowed we wouldn't have another dog, but then we all felt a great need for a canine companion so the search began. Mother telephoned and visited the local RSPCA dogs' home and chose a stray dog, but inevitably its rightful owner claimed it after a few days. We decided to go to a local animal sanctuary. My godmother, Auntie Kathleen, who was one of my

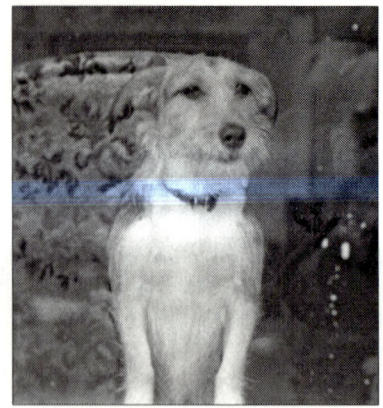

Suki

parents' church friends from Luton and bridesmaid at their wedding, was staying with us. She and her late husband, Stuart Weston who had worked at Mount Pleasant Post Office in London all his life, were both my godparents, and their daughter, Rosemary, and I still exchange cards and news at Christmas. We all went off to Wythall Animal Sanctuary, near Birmingham, where we found an odd assortment of birds, a one legged goat, donkeys and numerous dogs. We were shut in an enclosure and invited to inspect the animals. I saw a tiny face with big brown eyes peeping out of a kennel and that was it: I knew we had to give that dog a home. So Suki, as I named her, became our next family pet and companion. I maintain that as she had been neglected, she was so thankful for a loving home that she tried to make up with her affection. Her eyes told all, as did her tail, and she would carry on conversations using her tail; she didn't need to speak as her communication by other means was so efficient.

Work and School

IN MY TEENAGE years I did various jobs to earn extra pocket money. One of these was deputising for Gillian as a dental assistant at a practice overlooking the Heath. We acted as receptionist and helper, including mixing the fillings, which made us feel very important. My own regular job was babysitting, and I was kept busy helping Mrs Caragh Hanning and her husband Hugh with their young son, James. I started looking after James when he was a few months old until he was a toddler. At first they lived in a flat overlooking the Heath, but then moved to a larger house near the village. Hugh was a very successful journalist writing mainly about political, humanitarian and church affairs, and Caragh supported him at his London office. During the holidays I would look after James for the day, taking him for walks, often home to see Mother. Other days I helped with the housework. I grew very fond of the family and we still exchange Christmas cards. When I was in King's College Hospital as a patient Mrs Hanning visited me, and we played brain-teasing games of Scrabble, which took my mind off treatment. I also baby-sat for friends of the Hannings and once watched a 'Son et Lumiere' performance of Greenwich from a window of their home in Vanburgh Hill, a first class seat for such an occasion; and the baby slept throughout.

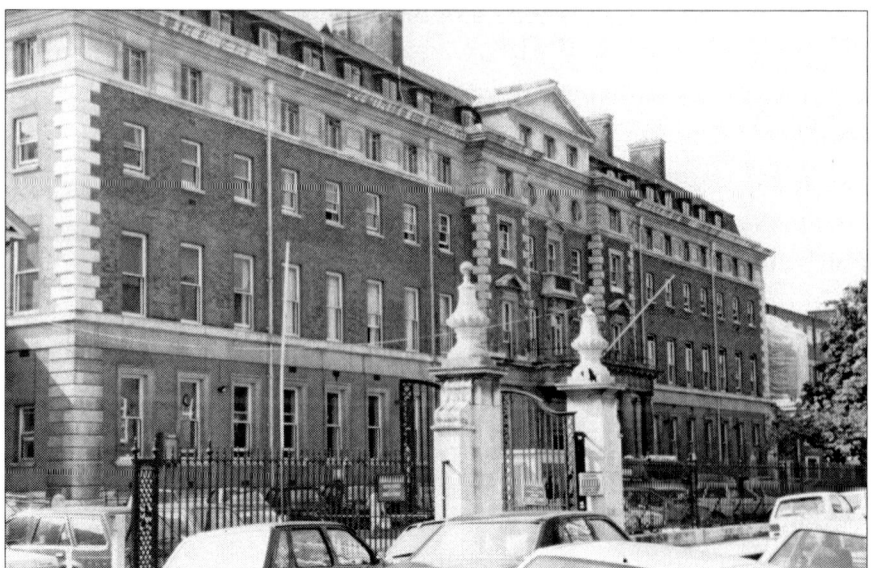

The front of King's College Hospital which became very familiar over the years

I had many friends at school, but Gillian (née Boyd) was my closest. We usually sat together and delighted in answering 'yes' when Gill/Jill was called out for registers, etc. We were part of a gang of six and I have kept in touch with Gillian and Prudence (née Green); it was a great pleasure to meet again Dorothy (née Parsons), another member of the gang, a few years ago and I hope the network will grow. Gillian and I lived near each other and I would call for her on our way to school. As well as both enjoying sport and playing in school teams, we had similar interests of Guides, and later our careers. At 16, I was still undecided about a career; my teachers wanted me to concentrate on mathematics but I was anxious to work with children. Children's nursing was high on the list, but when told I would have to do general nursing first, my enthusiasm waned. I then became increasingly interested in physiotherapy. My teachers couldn't persuade me to continue with A level mathematics, so at 17 I left school a year before I could take up a place at physiotherapy school having been accepted by both St Thomas's Hospital and King's College Hospital. The physiotherapist sister of father's colleague Archdeacon Sands advised me to take the place at the latter, so in the intervening year I studied O level physics and chemistry which the physiotherapy principal at King's, Miss Evelyn Stewart, suggested would be helpful. I took a job as clerical assistant at the National Provident Institute for Mutual Life Assurance in Gracechurch Street, London and went to Woolwich Polytechnic to study physics one evening a week and chemistry on another. After eight months I obtained passes in both subjects and this certainly helped with my physiotherapy training.

Elisabeth had left school at 17 and having obtained a place to start nursing training at St Bartholomew's Hospital the following year, went to Sweden where she worked as a nanny. Her first job was in Gothenberg, then after a few months she moved to Stockholm. The family there spent weekends at their cottage on one of the nearby islands and Elisabeth had a wonderful time exploring the country and making friends. Meanwhile Petrena, after some indecision about a future career when she left school, started work in a local public library. She enjoyed the work so much that she studied librarianship by correspondence courses, gaining membership of the Association after some years of study.

Holidays

During our Blackheath days, holidays were usually locums for Father; however one year Benedicta Whistler, a good friend who lived in the Paragon, Blackheath found us a holiday cottage in Battle, Sussex, where she had a family home. My father first met Benedicta at All Saint's church and learnt that she also worked for the church. When her mother visited Blackheath my mother would call at the Paragon and our family had a long friendship until Benedicta died in 2000. The cottage in Battle was very old and my parents had a four poster bed; we enjoyed getting into bed with them and drawing the curtains. My bedroom was on the top floor and was shaped like a ridge tent with sloping ceilings. That year we had a heatwave and I had to meet Father's unmarried sister, Auntie Margaret, from the train at Battle embalmed in calamine lotion as we had got very sunburnt. She was the oldest of my paternal grandparents' four children; two boys and two girls. They lived in Basingstoke where grandfather was Headmaster of St John's School until he died at an early age from tuberculosis, as did his younger daughter, Yvonne. The family then moved to Luton, when Father, the youngest, was four, to live with granny's sister. Granny had to work to support the family and was determined the boys would have a good education. She was rewarded as Father's older brother, Roland, and Father succeeded and were both awarded degrees at Cambridge; Roland at Selwyn College, and Father at Queen's College. Auntie Margaret worked from an early age at a hat factory in Luton, to help support the boys; later she looked after Roland's three children when his first wife, Thelma, died after childbirth. Five

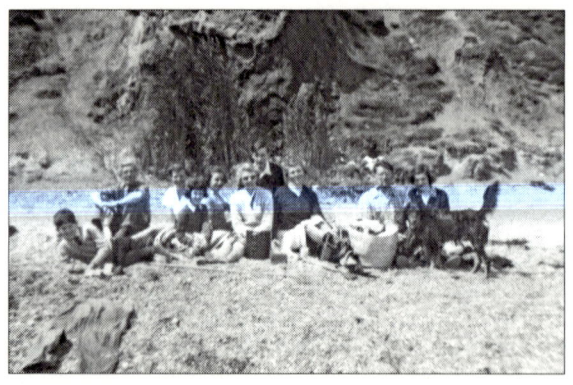

The Brown family, including cousins, and Aunt Margaret on holiday

years later when he married Ruth, she went back to work and was a school matron, first at St Alban's Girl's school, then at Abbots Bromley school and finally for Dr Barnado's at their boarding houses for The Princess Margaret School in Woodford Bridge, Essex. Having no home of her own after Granny died, she spent her holidays with Roland or us and when we lived in Blackheath she often visited on her days off.

The following years we had many happy visits to Suffolk and Norfolk, as well as occasional holidays in other parts of the country. When summer approached, Father drew a radius of 80 miles around Blackheath and then studied the *Church Times* for locums required within that area. We had, of necessity, very second hand cars, which unfortunately were liable to break down, so Father resolved to stay within their capability. The old tin trunk would be packed with essentials for the family of five plus dog, and that would be strapped on the rear of first 'No Joke' (our Austin 7), then later models which weren't much of an improvement in size or reliability. Two years running when I was about nine and ten we went to Huntingfield in Suffolk. The Rectory was huge with a vast garden which contained a veritable

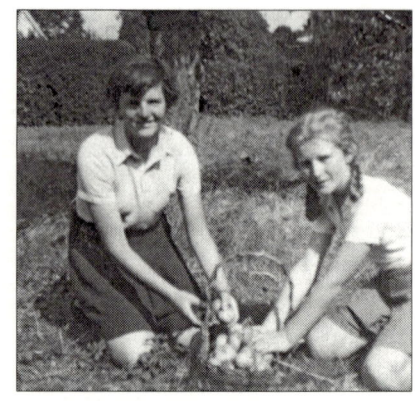

Elisabeth with Jill collecting fallen apples at Huntingfield

harvest of tomatoes and apples. The churchwarden, in his nineties but very active, insisted I accept a beautiful silver bangle with a gold leaf, which I still have. The church had a magnificent painted ceiling and I wondered how anyone could lie up there painting the roof, when I, sitting down at an easel, couldn't even make a flower look real.

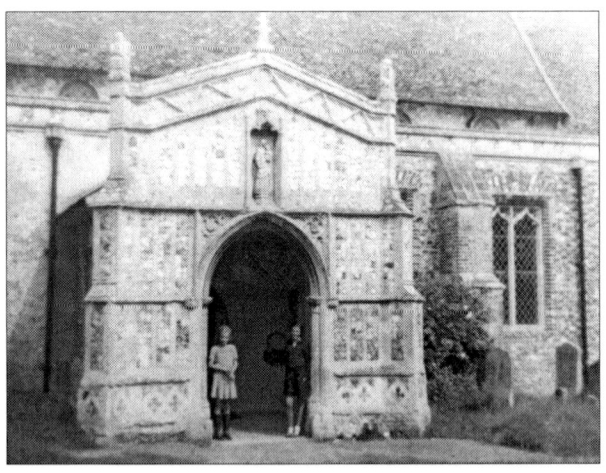

Petrena and Jill at the porch of of Huntingfield Church, Suffolk

Huntingfield was within reach of the sea, and we often went to Walberswick, which we christened 'Walziwigg', and which, though much gentrified, I gather is still much as it was in the early 1950s, with a small green and long main village street. There was a favourite fish and chip shop to which we walked for lunch if we hadn't taken sandwiches, which tended to become full of sand from the huge sand dunes with prickly Marram grasses – very painful for bare feet. When our Brown cousins joined us, those who were old enough clambered on the car running boards when we took the track down to the beach. We shared the task of going to fetch ice creams after lunch; when the wind blew, as it frequently did on the East

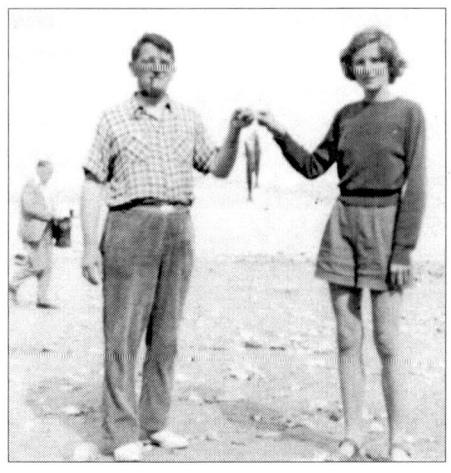

Jill and her father showing their catch after fishing for mackerel

Coast, they too would be coated in sand. Other days we walked along the dykes by the river and marshes separating Walberswick from Southwold.

We also had holidays with Uncle Roland and his wife, Ruth, and family, who lived at Grasmere. They had six children in all, a daughter, Sue who was much the same age as Elisabeth, and then twins Michael and Judy who were near Petrena's age, from his first marriage to Thelma; then with Ruth a son, Christopher, who was a little younger than me, followed by twins, Jenny and Timothy. Roland had been a teacher at Christ's Hospital school in Horsham, Sussex, but moved to be His Majesty's Inspector of Schools in the Lake District. Their house in Grasmere had an extensive garden going down to the lake, where we would swim and row over to the island with its goats, always friendly and keen to nibble any picnic food, or clothes. We went to the rush bearing festival, having decorated the young twins' pushchair which Aunt Ruth took in the procession. Another excitement

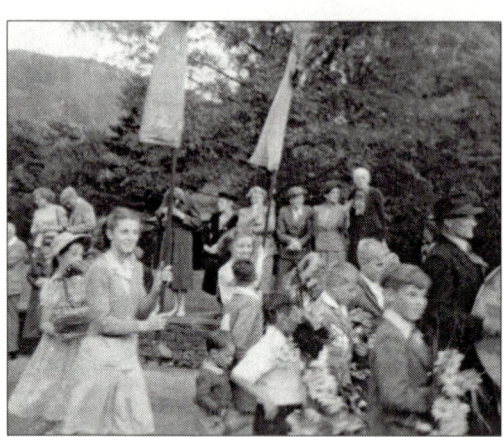

Cousin Sue carrying a banner in the procession at the Rush bearing Festival at Grasmere

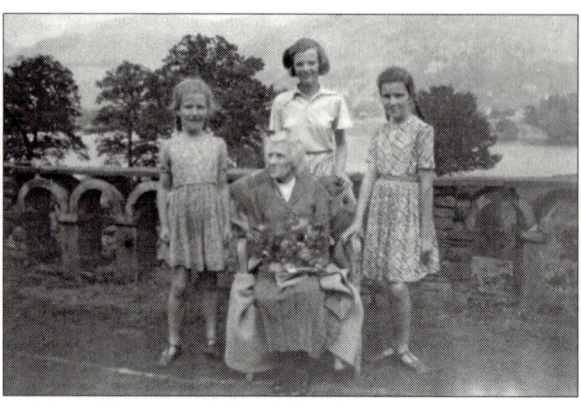

Granny Brown with Elisabeth, Petrena and Jill by Grasmere Lake

was the Grasmere games and standing in the field waiting anxiously for the hounds to come back from their mountain chase. We went walking in the mountains though I was only allowed on the gentle walks, as I was considered too young for serious climbs; Striding Edge was out of bounds.

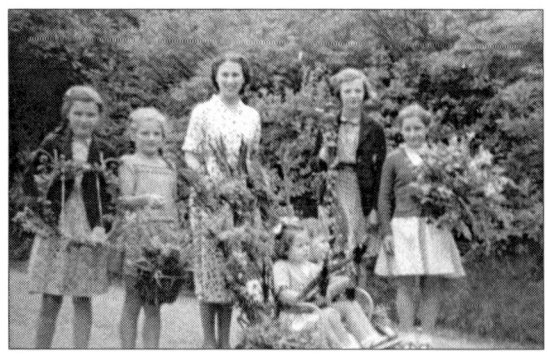

Aunt Ruth pushing twins Tim and Jenny, escorted by Elisabeth and Judy on the right and Petrena and Jill on the left at the Grasmere Rush bearing Festival

When I was 10 Auntie Margaret took me as her companion to Eastbourne for an Easter break, where we stayed in a guesthouse, and I was thoroughly spoilt. I had never stayed in a hotel or guesthouse before, nor been taken away as the only child. We went on buses to Beachy Head and the bays along the coast, as well as walking on the Promenade and listening to the band. I think we went for two years, but then heard that the Speakmans, who owned the guesthouse, had sold up.

I must have been 12 or so when Petrena and I went to North Devon with Mrs Pichler and her children to a hotel owned by friends of hers. We played 'Pooh sticks' from a tiny wooden bridge over the stream in the woods. Nearby was Hartland village, and when I visited that area in the 1980s it seemed little changed; I was delighted to see a board advertising 'Fosfelle', the hotel where we had stayed so many years before.

In the mid '50s we had teenagers from a Swedish scouting family staying with us; the family had given Father accommodation when he went to represent the British Scout Movement at a 'Duty to God' Scout Conference in Sweden, and they came on holidays with us. Karen, the eldest daughter, was older than me but we got on well;

her English was impeccable and she became one of the family. At the rectory in Stiffkey in Norfolk we were all reduced to uncontrollable laughter at the sight of her lying on the bed she had chosen; it was like a hammock and she was hidden in a dip in the middle. There was table tennis in the basement and one of the village lads who 'fancied ' Karen invited himself to come and have a game with us most evenings; Karen however was not amused and remained aloof.

When her brother, Lars, visited us another year we were staying at Easton in Suffolk. We watched in horror as Lars, riding the vicarage horse, was almost decapitated when the horse, out of control, galloped straight towards its stable. When mounted, Lars was a good eighteen inches too tall to get through the stable door, but being a strong lad he was able to hang on to the top doorframe while the horse got into its stable. When Elisabeth's French friend, Denise, came to stay in Blackheath, she seemed very aloof and disinterested in 'little sisters', and used to hurry to her bedroom where she had a collection of cheese labels. In those days people ate individual, small, boxed cheeses like Dairylea and Swiss Knight, which had their own distinctive decorative labels. These Denise collected and mounted in albums which she kept in the chest of drawers. The bedroom smelt of cheese after her visit and we had to leave the drawers in the garden for days to clear the smell. I had French and German penfriends, but as I was never a linguist our exchange of letters became more erratic until it ceased, and we never got to the stage of making exchange visits.

Health

So my childhood passed very happily. I think I was well-adjusted, lively and pretty healthy and of average ability. I don't remember the first general practitioner (GP) who delivered me into the world, Dr Jimmy Ross, but I met him on later visits to Welwyn Garden City. After my parents' deaths I continued our Christmas exchange of letters until he and then his wife Frances died. When I was a patient at King's College Hospital during the 1980s I met a Dr Euan Ross. I was asked to help with the medical student examinations which were being held on the ward, and acted as timekeeper and messenger for the practical examiners, for which I was paid. Dr Ross was one of these and turned out to be the son of Dr Jimmy.

When I was about eight I had measles and hid under the bedclothes from Dr Miller our GP and shot from one end of the bed to the other to avoid him, until he stripped the bedclothes; he must have thought me a very silly child. In 1951 my fingers got trapped in the train door and I nursed sore fingers for some weeks afterwards. During my teens I began to have more serious medical problems and was referred to the endocrine clinic at Guy's Hospital where I was found to have a deficiency of the hormone oestrogen. I was prescribed an early form of hormone replacement therapy. I also had what was then called 'growing pains' in my legs, and was very tall and lanky, for which I had regular x-rays to check my bone growth. My friends called me a 'dustbin' because I could always be relied on to finish up leftovers from any meal, and yet remained slim. From that time on my medical saga has developed as described in later chapters.

2

Office Junior in London

So FROM THE sheltered environment of a girls' public school to work in the big City of London early in September 1958. I felt very shy, and apart from knowing that my job description was 'clerical work and general office duties' I had no idea what lay in store. I wondered what I could wear, for I had a very limited wardrobe and I didn't know what was expected of me. My parents managed on a very meagre income in those war and immediate post-war days and with three girls and only one wage earner, we didn't have many clothes. So Mother and I visited the shops in Lewisham, a bus ride away, to buy some 'tidy' work clothes to set me up initially. For work I walked to Blackheath station where I took the train to London Bridge, familiar from visits to Southwark Cathedral, but I wasn't used to the rush hour, which even in 1958-59 was quite a crush.

The short walk over London Bridge where one could observe movements of boats in the Pool of London, past the Monument brought me to the National Provident Institute for Mutual Life Assurance, (NPI), on the corner of Gracechurch Street. However the office was to be demolished within the year and we would move to another nearby building.

My duties were to open the mail every morning, distribute to the appropriate person in our department, answer the straightforward letters, and sort out the cheques for claims. There was often a very tense and busy half-hour at the end of each day when I had to collect the letters and put the cheques in the correct envelopes before they could be signed by my boss, and posted. My financial experience had been limited to pocket money, then shopping expenses and I was amazed to handle cheques for large sums of money such as £20,000 and more.

There were five staff in our department and I was the 'general dogsbody' for them all. This included one very important daily task: to get their orders for lunchtime snacks. We were issued with luncheon vouchers and I had to collect these with each person's requirements, then go to the local baker to buy various filled rolls and sandwiches; light relief from the office routine and I didn't mind. I was responsible for getting the clients' dusty folders out for the more senior staff to deal with, and this meant a walk or ride to the basement in the rickety lift. It was bad enough when the office building was standing but after demolition had started and only the shell was left, it was very scary going to the basement in the creaking and groaning machine. The lift porter was a very large gentleman called Jimmy who was helpful to us young employees advising us, on occasion, about the senior staff whims; he would operate the lift for me if he could when I had to fetch the folders.

During lunch breaks I would have something to eat from one of the local restaurants, such as the Kahawa, Jo Lyons, Jolly's, the Express Dairy, and would then explore the Monument area. Occasionally I would venture as far as St Paul's Cathedral but that was rather a rush. I continued to attend the Endocrine Clinic at Guy's hospital and an operation was suggested but not carried out. I had several boy friends from the office during the year; also from the squash club in Blackheath where we played regularly. Peter from the latter took me to concerts at Goldsmith's College. We also went out for a meal from time to time and to some dances, but dancing was never my strong point. John worked in London and this friendship continued when I moved to live and work in Liverpool, before our ways parted. Imagine my surprise on recognising one of my office colleagues in Salisbury market some 30 years later! By then I was using a wheelchair and that rather confused him, but his face hadn't changed and nor apparently had mine. One of the more senior staff also appeared in Salisbury, and I learnt that several people from the NPI had moved there when Friends' Provident built new offices.

I was in the netball team for the NPI and we played other offices at various venues. I didn't disclose that I had a physiotherapy place at King's for the following year, nor that I was studying physics and chemistry to GCE level at Woolwich Polytechnic after work, but there was no great surprise when I gave in my notice. I have never regretted that year in the City for it taught me a great deal about life in the big world outside school, and prepared me for meeting and communicating with the general public.

My social life revolved round my home and family. Several of my friends were still studying at the High School so I continued to see them regularly, and Gillian and I played squash and tennis. Elisabeth was engaged to be married to Brian Ward-Lilley and we often went to Brian's parents' home in Eltham, to play tennis. My mother had been a keen player for many years so she encouraged us and was pleased to see my enthusiasm and successes. As I was keen to save as much money as I could, to fund my physiotherapy training,

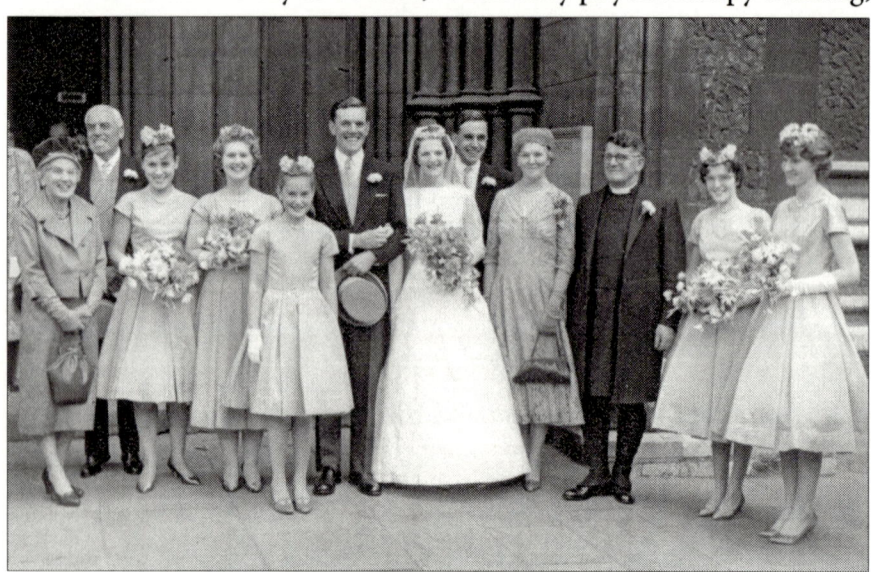

Elisabeth and Brian with their families and bridesmaids on the steps of Southwark Cathedral after their wedding.

I continued baby-sitting for the Hannings and friends. I did physics and chemistry homework when my young charges were asleep and passed both exams before I went to King's.

Elisabeth was now a qualified nurse, having trained at St Bartholomew's Hospital and we went to the Christmas Carols at the Church of St.Bartholomew the Great when she was in the choir. She met Brian at a friend's party and after they were engaged took a job as theatre staff nurse at Eltham and Mottingham Cottage Hospital. They had found a flat nearby, convenient for Elisabeth's work and Brian's office in London and planned to get married. Petrena and I were asked to be bridesmaids together with two of Elisabeth's best friends and Mary Pichler. Auntie Margaret made our burnt apricot dresses, and I went to Woodford Bridge, where she was house mother at the Princess Margaret School, for fittings. Shoes were dyed to match the dress and I am horrified at the stiletto heels we wore for the occasion. The service took place at Southwark Cathedral on 5th September 1959 shortly before I started my training. George Reindorp, the Provost, took the service. We changed into our dresses at the Reindorp's house on the South Bank and drove to the Cathedral along the narrow riverside streets. Afterwards we walked in procession through the Borough Market and over Borough High Street to St Thomas' Street where my parents had organised the wedding reception in the Chapter House. A policeman held up the traffic to allow us to cross the busy road. (When we moved to Salisbury in 1977 we renewed our friendship with George, as he was now the Bishop. He invited Father to become Priest in Charge of Odstock, Nunton and Bodenham, when he retired as Bishop of Birmingham.)

At the time Father was secretary of the South London Church Fund, Vice Provost of Southwark Cathedral and Archdeacon of Lewisham. His preaching duties took him around the Southwark Diocese and in particular to the parishes in his Archdeaconry, so he was busy at weekends, at the office during the week, and with evening meetings.

✳ *Walking on Wheels* ✳

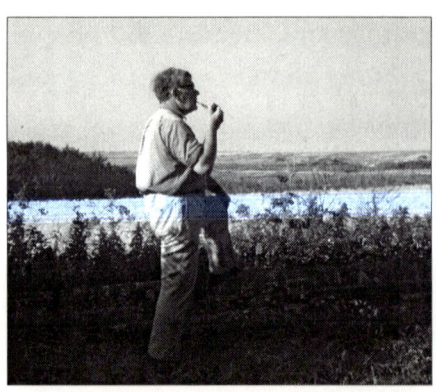
Father contemplating the view in Suffolk

We had a holiday in Suffolk during August of that year, at a tiny cottage at Wenhaston. The first weekend we discovered that the power cut and a strange smell permeating the cottage were both caused by a dead mouse behind the cooker. We visited the small villages in mid-Suffolk and also explored the coast, bathed regularly in the sea and enjoyed a relaxing couple of weeks. I then had another week with my parents by the sea in Norfolk before starting at King's.

3
To King's

After the excitement of the wedding, the next major event in my life was the start of three year's training in October 1959 at King's College Hospital Physiotherapy School, so I had to get myself ready and buy the recommended textbooks and uniform. I travelled by train from Blackheath to Denmark Hill, on the Victoria line changing at Lewisham. There weren't many trains and timing was critical; sometimes there was an anxious wait at Lewisham. Fortunately there was another student from King's making the same journey, so I had moral support as she was an experienced commuter. Train strikes seemed a fairly regular occurrence in those days, so then we had to go by bus which took a very long time, or even by bicycle.

There were some five daygirls in our set of 16; the others lived in the student hostel at Herne Hill for the first six months and then moved to flats of their choice for the remainder of their training. The daygirls tended to stick together, but we were a happy set, and all friendly and supportive towards each other. I am still in contact with 12 of the set and we now meet regularly though as travelling is difficult for me, the reunions are usually held in Salisbury.

We were measured for our uniforms and until fairly recently I had one of the green aertex shirts that we wore for some of the lectures and gym classes, and my green blazer with its King's crest. We wore white serge overalls and white caps, which had to be starched, then folded exactly, which really served no useful purpose as far as we

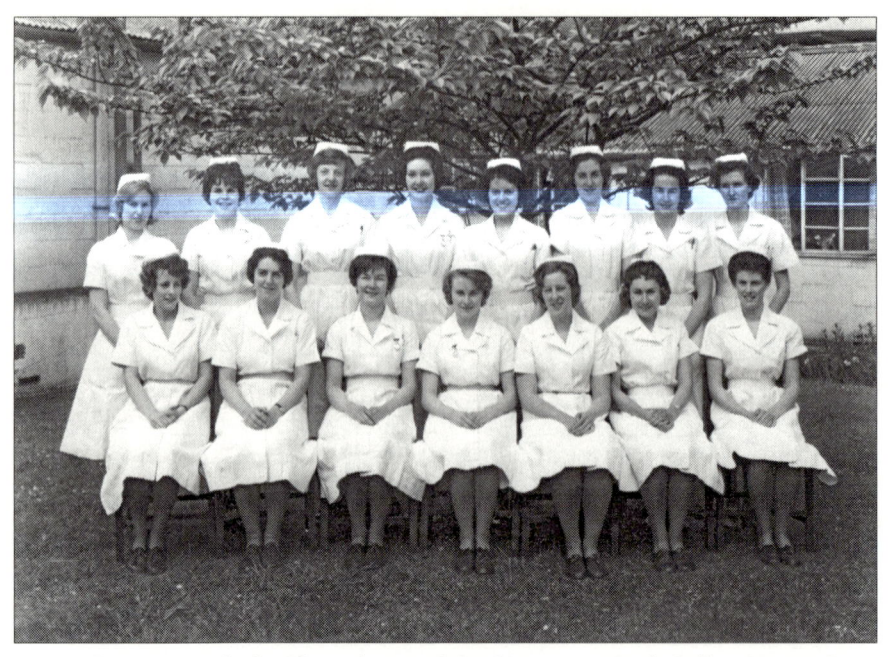

Our set outside the Physiotherapy School rooms at King's College Hospital, September 1959

could see. A black canvas belt and black lace-up shoes completed our uniform when wearing the white overall; grey woollen, divided skirts with gym shoes with the green shirt.

The Physiotherapy School was very small at that time and in a prefabricated building between two of the hospital wards. After I left, a new department was built, and later a combined physiotherapy and nursing school called Normanby College. Our lectures took place in one of the classrooms, our practical sessions in another designated room, and exercise classes in the gymnasium. Miss Evelyn Stewart, the Principal, and the staff also had small rooms, and there was a small library. There was no common room so for lunch we would go either to the canteen or more usually to 'Emmies'. Emmie was a lovely, rotund lady who sold cheese rolls, coffee and biscuits in one of the houses near the hospital. These buildings have disappeared: the new Dental School was built on the site of Emmies and physiotherapy students now take a degree course at King's College in the Strand.

For the first six months we had lectures, practical exercise classes and practical electrical sessions. We had to learn the basic anatomy of the whole body, physiology, electrotherapy (treatment by electrical means), and the basic medical and surgical conditions we would encounter when we started treatments. We were all required to be models for the final examinations in physiotherapy and that gave us some insight into what would be expected of us at the end of our training. Each set had a weekly rota for 'class monitor' who had to collect essays from the whole set, and wash lint pads used in electrotherapy practical sessions; no one liked their week of duty. It was a busy six months with regular essays to write and preliminary examinations at the end. Failure meant serious consideration whether you should continue with training, and two of our set were advised to leave.

I had worked hard and studied at home, as I enjoyed the subjects and found them fascinating. On my father's death in 1994 I had to dispose of his papers and found a letter written after the examinations by the Principal to him saying that my examination results were 'among the best we have had in the school for a long time' and that my practical work was up to standard; I was 'observant and careful and as she shows understanding well above average, I am quite sure that as she gains confidence she will develop into an excellent physiotherapist'; I was shy and quiet but the School were pleased to have me.

We returned after the Easter holidays to work for three weeks on a ward doing basic nursing duties, including some nights, before treating patients by physiotherapy. I stayed at the hostel, as it was impractical to travel to and from Blackheath. We were allowed to state our ward preference and I asked for and was allocated to Princess Elizabeth, the childrens' ward, and was very happy to be working with children. I watched my first operation with great trepidation but was so interested in what was going on that I didn't feel in the least bit shaky. I became very involved with my small patients even in that short time, and was sad when we had a death on the ward; my Christian faith taught me to cope with that and with other bereavements over the years.

The days that followed were divided into lectures and treating patients. At first it seemed daunting but we were well prepared and supervised by qualified staff for the first months. We rotated around out-patients, the gym, clinics, and wards which gave us experience of the various specialties. My first stint was in out-patients where I took classes, as well as having individual patients.

I continued to travel by train to King's and often had companions, either from the hospital or friends in Blackheath. By this time we were settling into groups in our set: I often travelled with Pat Waite who lived in Greenwich, but my particular friend was another Pat, Dee, who lived in Sydenham. Playing squash at the Priory club with Gillian Boyd at weekends, we compared our work as she was studying physiotherapy at Guy's.

We had plenty of visitors at home: Elisabeth and Brian from their Eltham home, Auntie Margaret and Mother's only relative Auntie Florrie. In July 1960 my parents celebrated their 25th wedding anniversary with a family party at the Strand Palace Hotel, followed by a visit to a ballet at the Festival Hall.

Soon after this Father was invited to be Bishop of Warrington in Lancashire, Suffragan to the Bishop of Liverpool, Clifford Martin.

Church attendance was entirely voluntary but from an early age it became part of my life

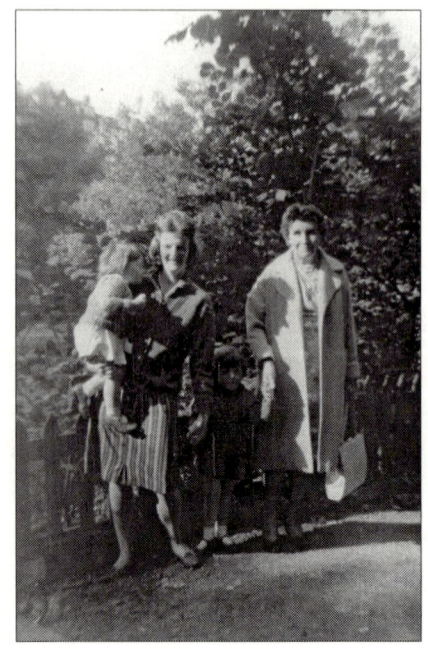

Auntie Florrie with Elisabeth and Sarah

and I either worshipped at our parish church or Southwark Cathedral. When at King's I went to the hospital chapel; I found it very peaceful and later when a patient I went there regularly to find tranquillity and solace.

At King's we had split holidays, so that half the students would be away at one time; when it was my turn I went with my parents first to Dorset and then on to Liverpool. We stayed in a well-equipped second floor flat in an attractive Dorset village called Sydling St Nicholas. The owner of the house lived on the ground floor and generously allowed clergy families to holiday in her upstairs rooms. This was an ideal base to explore Dorset and to visit Uncle Roland and his family who had moved from the Lake District to nearby Dorchester. Then we drove north to Stafford where we stayed overnight with the late Dudley and Marjorie Hodges. Father had trained for the Ministry with him at Cuddesdon and both spent time at the Church of St John the Divine, Kennington. When we were in Blackheath, Dudley was vicar of a church in Eltham, and parish priest for my brother-in-law's family. After our move to Liverpool we would regularly stop in Stafford with them when travelling to and from London. Later they moved to Lichfield, where he was Precentor of the Cathedral at the time we went to Birmingham, and then retired to Salisbury where we also eventually found a house.

At Liverpool we went to see our future home in the West Derby area, 'quite a nice area', I recorded and the house 'enormous with a vast garden'. There we met a Diocesan representative, Mr.Straw, who took us to the Royal Hotel, then a highly ranked establishment. The date of Father's Consecration at York Minster, was to be 30th November 1960, St Andrews Day.

We returned to College on September 11th and I went to see various flats and rooms near King's, but didn't find anything I liked. Then I had an offer to live with the Bishop of Woolwich, John Robinson and his wife who lived at 17 Manor Way, Blackheath Park with their four young children. I moved in on 16th November, the day before my family moved north.

During the term I was plagued by acne which bothered me greatly and by my hormone problems, so I was referred back to Guy's Hospital. I had ultra-violet irradiation from one of the senior students at King's for my skin, which responded well. We started lectures and later dissections with a professor at King's College in the Strand. After initial concern about dealing with corpses I found the sessions interesting and relevant; preliminary exams, which we would take the following May, included anatomy and physiology papers. Seeing the actual bones and muscles in position was extremely helpful as I have a photographic memory. I did well in the mock exams but was told that I was still shy and lacked confidence, traits that I have tried to overcome for most of my life, and hopefully are now improved. I particularly enjoyed working with children at the special school at Thurlow Park and at the Belgrave Children's Hospital. I also had some weeks at the hydrotherapy pool, and at occupational therapy where I helped make various gadgets under supervision.

On 29th November I travelled with Elisabeth and Brian to York for Father's Consecration. The day was chilly, grey and wet and the Minster very cold. Nineteen

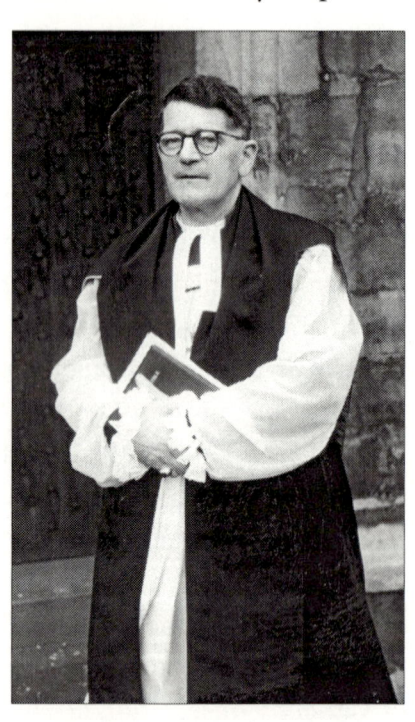

Father after his Consecration as a Bishop outside York Minster

Bishops were present and the service was memorable for its dignity, also colour from the numerous clergy in their decorated ecclesiastical robes. I noted that the singing was 'fairly good' – obviously not up to Southwark Cathedral standard in my opinion. Lunch was provided after the Service and I then returned to London by car with a friend of Father's. I arrived back at Manor Way past midnight and went to College the next morning.

Elisabeth and her husband soon moved north: in December they left for Norton near Stockton on Tees, where Brian had a job working for ICI. Auntie Margaret joined my parents in May 1961 when she retired; before this she welcomed me to stay with her at Woodford Bridge. The Pichlers were still in Kidbrooke Grove, Blackheath, and the Robinsons were most kind to me. The squash club was only five minutes walk from their house, so a very convenient place to meet my friends. In December my GP referred me back to the endocrinologist at Guy's and an appointment was made for the New Year.

I was very excited when the end of term came and I travelled by train to Liverpool to see my new home, looking more familiar with our furnishings. My parents and Petrena showed me some of the City that first holiday and we attended the magnificent, lofty Anglican Cathedral, which was not yet completed, and experienced some of the traditional Christmas services. The processions were magnificent, with the clergy and choir dressed in emerald green robes which contrasted well with the sandstone bricks of the building, all very different from the historical Cathedral of Southwark.

So a new chapter in my life began.

4
Working towards Qualification ~ 1961

WHAT A MOVE, from London where I had spent all my schooldays, to Liverpool. My parents persuaded me to have a break during the Christmas holiday as they knew I was working hard at King's. West Derby, the suburb we had moved to, was a mixture of large private houses, smaller homes and high rise flats, several churches, pubs and local shops. The parish church, St Mary's, in an area known as 'the village' was next to a magnificent gated entrance to Croxteth Park; we enjoyed many a walk through the estate on the pedestrian only, tarmac road. On this and other walks we missed Andy, our dog, who died shortly before we moved north. Liverpool is well served with parks which form an almost unbroken semicircle around the suburbs, the river Mersey and coastal paths of Crosby completing the circle.

I explored West Derby and the nearby suburb of Knotty Ash by bicycle, which was pleasant as apart from steep hills down to the city

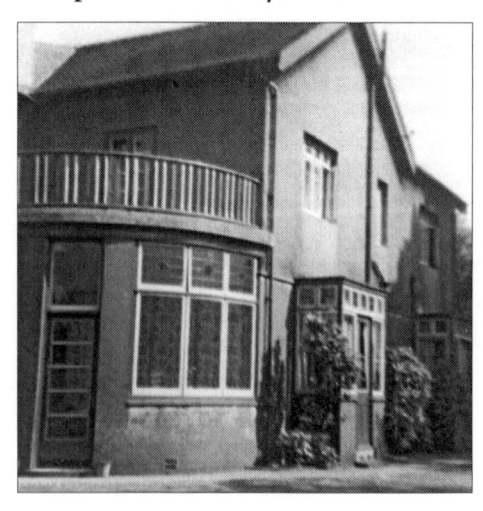

A view of St Martin's, Sandfield Park, our Liverpool home

✳ *Working towards Qualification* ✳

centre Liverpool is flat. Mother and I went to the busy city centre by bus and gradually I learnt my way round the shopping area and galleries. Later I got to know the older parts of the city, housing numerous offices and the seafarer's church of St Nicholas, near the docks and ferry to New Brighton. At first I found it difficult to understand the Liverpool accent, known as

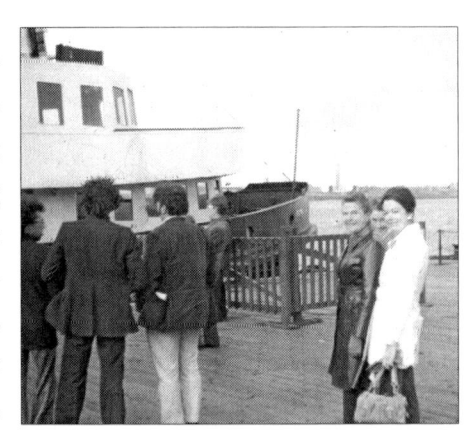

Doris and Hazel Kabity going aboard the Mersey ferry (Hazel far right)

'scouse', as not only do Liverpudlians have a distinctive accent but a local vocabulary; our daily help, Annie, who spoke with a very broad accent, was a helpful interpreter.

At Christmas and New Year we attended several church services and I was proud to see Father dressed in his splendid Bishop's robes. Elisabeth and Brian joined us for part of the holiday and we climbed up the tower of the Cathedral, where we had a panoramic view of the city and across the Mersey to Birkenhead and the Wirral area of Cheshire. We drove to Crosby, the mouth of the river Mersey, for a bracing walk on the beach: it was always windy there with the air rushing in from the Atlantic; little did we know that we would move to live in Great Crosby a couple of years later.

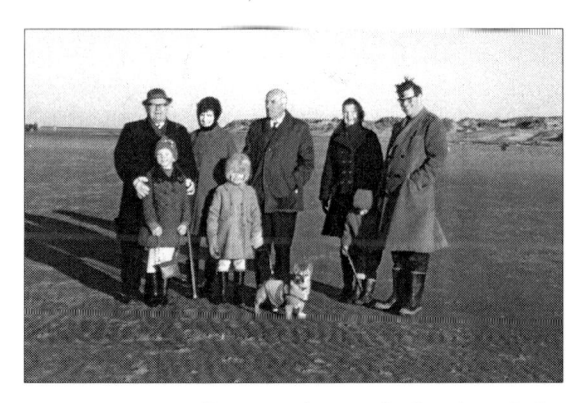

A New Year walk on windy Formby beach with dog Judy and Father with Sarah, Petrena with Rachel, Ken Ward-Lilley, Elisabeth and Brian

People were friendly and welcomed us: we went to Bishop Clifford Martin's home in Woolton where we met his charming wife, Margaret. Ann, his secretary, hearing I enjoyed music and singing, invited me to a party at her home and carol singing at one of Liverpool's hospitals.

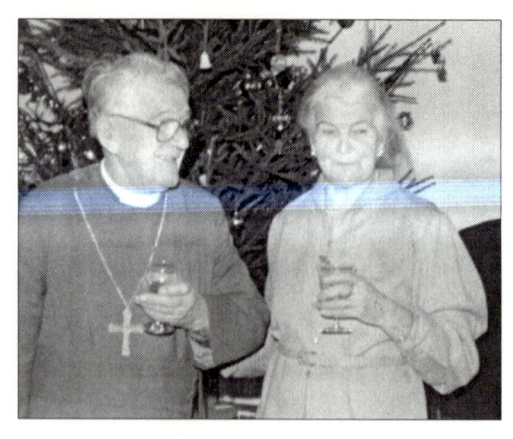

My parents who were so supportive

Before I returned to King's, we had our first visit to Liverpool Playhouse and saw *I Killed the Count* which was extremely funny. The theatre in the city centre was small but had good productions and we visited it many times during our nine years in Liverpool.

Our house was large, with plenty of spare rooms, and surrounded by thick hedges and bushes; it felt damp and was unsuitable. The garden was vast and included a four-car garage, two large greenhouses and

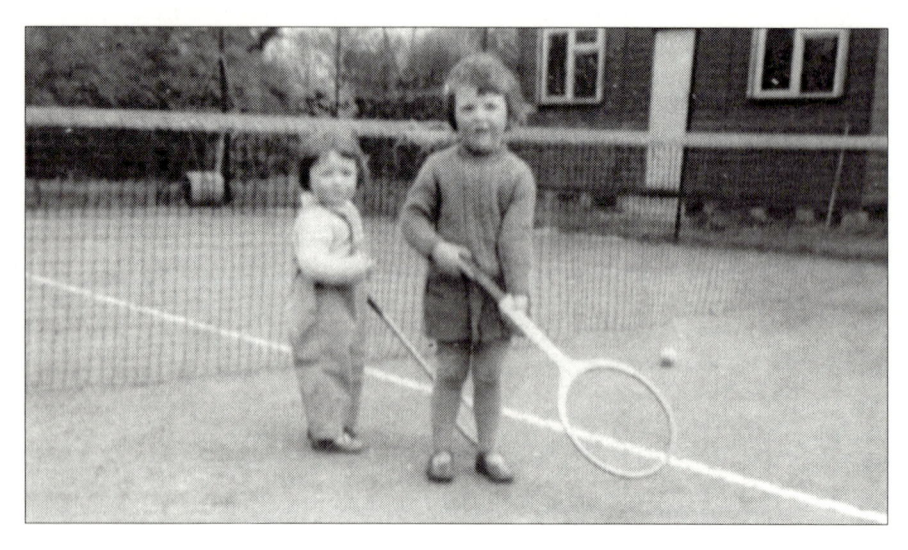

Sarah and Rachel playing on the tennis court at St Martin's.

a tennis court. Fortunately the tennis club at nearby St James Church used and maintained the court and we played at other times, but the whole garden was a liability; Father had little time for gardening and was never an enthusiast. After some months the diocesan surveyor examined the property and found serious structural problems. My parents were told that if they could find a more suitable property which the surveyor approved, the diocese would be prepared to buy it for the home of the Suffragan Bishop.

Back to London

AFTER TWO WEEKS' holiday I returned to London. The train was overcrowded and cold; the heating had failed, as it did regularly, making the journey seem very long. My first practical of the term was in the occupational therapy department: we needed to know how our therapy colleagues worked as many areas of our treatments overlapped. The second day of term I had an appointment at Guy's to see the endocrinologist Dr Bishop. My wrist and hip joints were X-rayed again as they had previously shown retardation of the epiphyses (a portion of bone attached to the main bone by cartilage, which becomes consolidated with it as growth ceases), and my hormone levels were still abnormal. I was concerned as my periods were very erratic but I was told not to worry until I married and wanted children. I was prescribed tablets to take before breakfast and told to drink a pint of milk a day to strengthen my bones.

In spring 1961, fees were due for the preliminary examination, part of our final qualification for the Chartered Society of Physiotherapy. Failure would mean a second fee for the retake and delay in qualification, and finances concerned us all. I had saved money from my work at the National Provident Institute and babysitting, and had a student grant from the London County Council (LCC), plus a small grant from a private foundation, the Thomas Wall Trust, but medical books were expensive and I had to watch my budget.

I studied most evenings and part of weekends but enjoyed the work and managed to gain reasonable marks for most of my essays. My second placement was in the gymnasium, taking classes or treating individual patients. Fortunately we had practised exercise classes with our fellow students as patients under the guidance of the tutor, Miss Jobson, but I preferred treating individual patients rather than taking classes.

Towards the end of term, one of our set, Susan Nepean, announced that she was leaving immediately to get married. We were surprised and sorry as she had become part of the team and was an able student. Twenty years later when I was living in Salisbury, she saw me on television taking part in a film about access for disabled people, and we renewed our friendship more strongly than when we were at King's, and have kept in touch for the past thirty years.

In contrast to the surrounding corridors and departments, the hospital chapel, situated in the very centre of the hospital, was a haven of peace. I regularly attended the lunch time services, or whenever I felt the need for some time of peace and reflection. Later when I was a patient I continued this practice.

In March 1961, I was surprised to receive a letter from Dr Bishop telling me to stop the medication he had prescribed and to return the drugs at my next appointment. Mother later said she had noticed deterioration in my health from that time. I developed a debilitating 'muscular rheumatism' that prevented me playing in a netball match for King's; I had to umpire instead and was also unable to play squash.

As the end of term approached, I realised I had been living away from home for four months. Bishop John and his wife, Ruth, were very welcoming though extremely busy; the four children, aged from three to ten were lively and intelligent. I looked after them on occasions, took them for walks and was invited to join some of their parties and activities. My bedsitting room, where I could entertain friends, was spacious but I joined the family for meals which Ruth prepared; the large kitchen had a long wooden table with bench seats parallel to the Aga; in winter we all wanted to sit nearest the heat. During the week I left the house at 8 am, returning at about 6 pm for the evening meal, then had a couple of hours studying, so there was little time for socialising. However at week-ends I met with friends and played squash; sometimes Bishop John challenged me to a game, until he damaged his back in a car accident. I was quite a good player because of my long arms and legs. My bicycle was used for getting about. All Saint's Church on Blackheath, where Father had helped, became my parish church. I visited the Pichlers or Gillian, and continued babysitting for my regular families.

Some weekends I spent at Woodford Bridge with Auntie Margaret, who missed her visits to Kidbrooke Grove. I missed my parents and Petrena too and regularly wrote them long letters. Father was a good correspondent, a trait which I have inherited, and he kept me up to date with life in Liverpool; Petrena sent me paperbacks for leisure reading. Elisabeth also wrote with news of her new home in Stockton on Tees; she and Brian were expecting their first child in April and I knitted baby clothes for her. Father came to London during term time for meetings that included Church Assembly and sometimes stayed at the Robinsons; it was good to see him but I was unhappy when he returned to Liverpool.

We completed the syllabus for the preliminary exams a week before the end of term. I was especially happy as my parents were coming to London for the Consecration of George Reindorp as Bishop of Guildford at Southwark Cathedral. I attended the service and later that day we drove home to Liverpool.

A Break in Liverpool

THE TWO WEEKS' holiday passed all too quickly and I was very happy being home with my family. We had a new addition: Judy, a two-year old Welsh corgi whom Mother, having missed a dog so much, got by answering an advertisement in the local paper. We loved her dearly and she was good company when exploring the neighbourhood on foot, but of all our dogs she was my least favoured as she was unpredictable.

With exams looming the following month, I made time for some revision but also enjoyed my first games of tennis on our court with Father and Petrena. On club night, members often invited us to have a game too, which was a good way of meeting new friends.

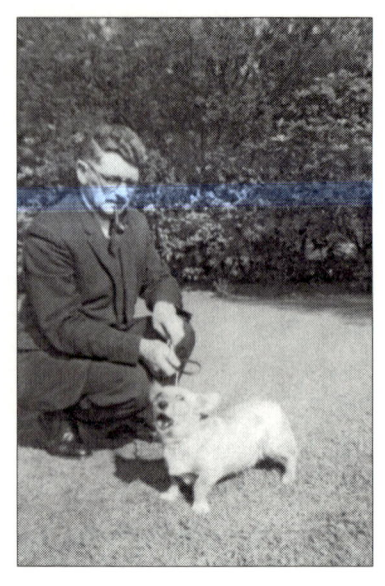

Father with dog Judy

Father had commitments in London so the final Sunday of my holiday he drove me back; I was upset and depressed about leaving the family. After a week, the Robinsons went on holiday and I stayed for a few days with the Pichlers before moving on to the Henkels. I was studying hard for the exams in early May: three written papers and a viva to be held at the Chartered Society of Physiotherapy buildings in Queen Square, London, to which Gillian and I travelled together.

I went home for my birthday during the Whitsun holiday, with Gillian and Marilla, both school friends. Marilla's father had offered to pay our first class train fares, a new experience for me. Unfortunately my viva came after the holiday, but I managed to enjoy the break and show my friends some of the sights of Liverpool.

Completion of exams coincided with the next rotation of duties; we were half way through our training and working towards the intermediate exam in twelve months' time, provided we had passed the preliminary exam. We were known as junior intermediates, having more responsibilities and treating patients with more complex

Working towards Qualification

conditions. Working on the obstetrics and gynaecology unit, I was invited to observe a birth; I found this quite wonderful and very relevant as Elisabeth had recently given birth to Sarah, my first niece. My next rotation was to the hydrotherapy department: the buoyancy and warmth of the water was most therapeutic and I learnt how to make use of these features in treatments.

I thoroughly enjoyed the theoretical and practical work and life at college, though I was still homesick and often found it hard to hold back tears when speaking to the family on the telephone, or when I met Father on his visits to London. My parents and Auntie Margaret were concerned and thought I was studying too hard; Father wrote to Miss Stewart, but I didn't know of this till 1994 when I found correspondence in which he had asked her if I could transfer to the Liverpool School of Physiotherapy. She replied that it would be a pity: I was doing well and my colleagues, although they sometimes teased me, were very fond of me; my theoretical work was of a very high

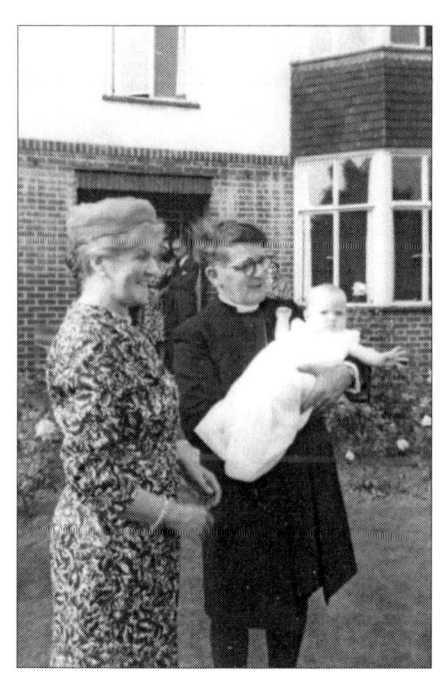

My parents at Sarah's Christening *Elisabeth and Brian with baby Sarah*

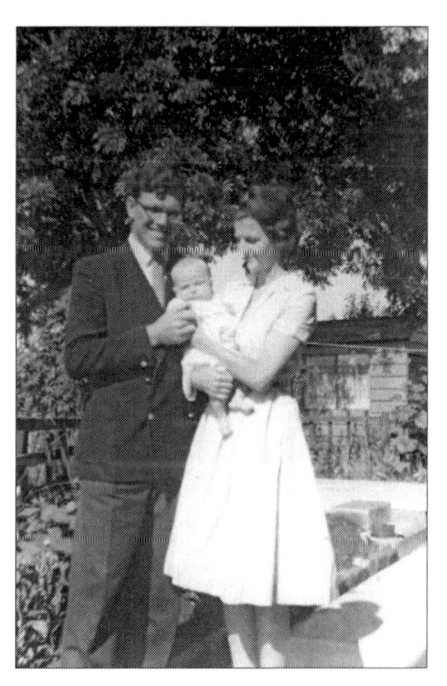

standard, and the staff considered my work with patients well up to standard.

I passed the Preliminary examination, and was nominated for the physiotherapy prize of the Southeast Region of the Chartered Society. A few weeks later I heard I was the winner and received a generous book token; I bought a *Blakiston's New Gould Medical Dictionary* to which I still refer. Having covered all the anatomy and physiology of the body during our first eighteen months, the final weeks of term concentrated on diseases and conditions we would be treating in the coming months.

My parents were staying in London early in July as Father had numerous meetings, and I saw them most evenings. Their visit culminated with the annual Lord Mayor of London's Banquet for Bishops at the Mansion House (which I was to attend the following year). My own social life had been busy: I played tennis and squash with local friends as well as with John, my boyfriend. One evening

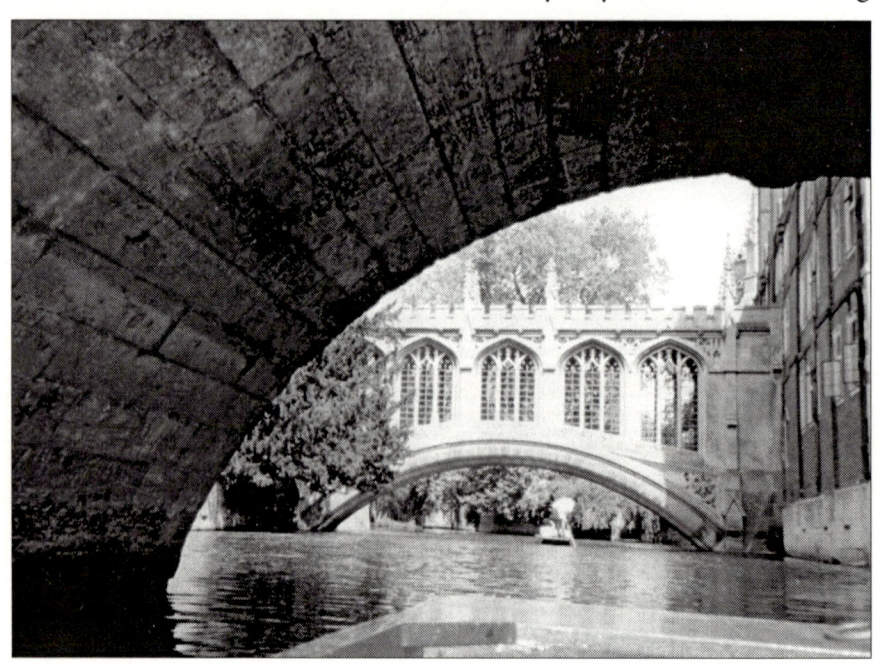

Punting on the River Cam

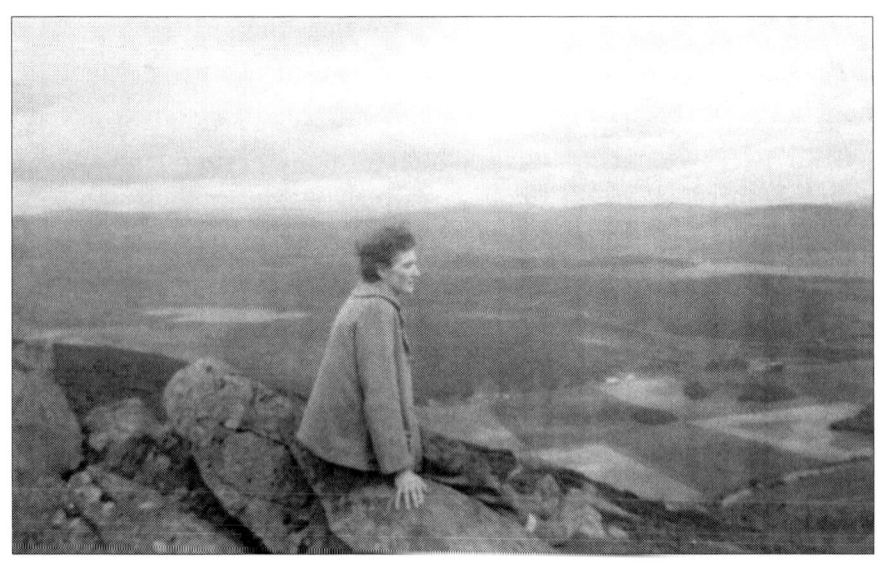

Jill, windswept, but admiring a view over the Scottish countryside

he took me to meet his parents and have dinner at their Petts Wood home, and another evening I had my first experience of an office dinner dance at a London restaurant. Bishop John was away lecturing in America so I babysat more for the Robinsons as well as for my regular families.

Auntie Margaret and I went to Cambridge to visit my cousin Michael, Roland's oldest son, who was reading geography at Selwyn College. The day was fine and we went punting on the river Cam; I was hopeless but fortunately Mike was more skilled. We also went to evensong at King's College; the beauty of the architecture and the singing of the choir overwhelmed me.

Summer Holiday

ONCE HOME IN Liverpool I started driving lessons with Father: I longed to drive and was saving for my own car.

Later we went to Forfar, Scotland where Father took a locum; he loved his parish duties. We walked miles in the hills and glens,

Glen Ceriog being a favourite. Glamis Castle with its superb paintings impressed us, and the quaint towns had their own fascination. Lunches were taken in pubs if we hadn't made a picnic. Several parishioners who were landed gentry 'wined and dined' us and we enjoyed gorgeous, fresh Scottish raspberries from their spacious gardens. Elisabeth, Brian, and Sarah joined us for our second week and I was thrilled to help care for my new niece; it was good to see the baby whom I had been knitting clothes for. The last weekend Petrena came for a brief visit.

Mary and Peter Pichler, our neighbours from Blackheath, visited us at home before I returned to King's They didn't know Liverpool at all, so we were able to show them some of the city.

King's Again

Returning to London for the final year of training I again stayed with the Henkels in Blackheath for two weeks as the Robinsons were away on holiday. Our set now worked with patients all day while the set above had their holiday. I was back in the pool until mid-day, and scheduled to return to Thurlow Park School for physically handicapped children for the rest of the day; I had greatly enjoyed the previous placement there. However the children were still on holiday, so I transferred to outpatients for the remainder of the working day. Life was more relaxed without lectures and essays, so I was able to see more of friends and play tennis and squash regularly, and also see John. Sarah was christened by Father at Eltham, and we had a family week-end party there which was great fun and a bonus for me.

When all the students returned from holiday we resumed our usual pattern of half a day treating patients and half a day of lectures, which covered more complex conditions and general medical knowledge. We practised massage and apparently mine felt more

※ *Working towards Qualification* ※

effective than it appeared to an observer. At this time I developed pain in first one shoulder and then the other. I did not disclose this in case it interrupted my training, and thankfully it disappeared by my resting as much as possible, but in retrospect this was probably a sign of the shoulder problems I developed later in life.

Weekends were busy and I visited Mother's cousin, Auntie Florrie, and her husband Bob in Luton, as well as local friends: Benedicta Whistler and the Pichlers, and Mrs McPhail and Auntie Millie, our former neighbours. The Pichlers moved to a small farm opposite Brands Hatch, Kent in late autumn 1961; fortunately there

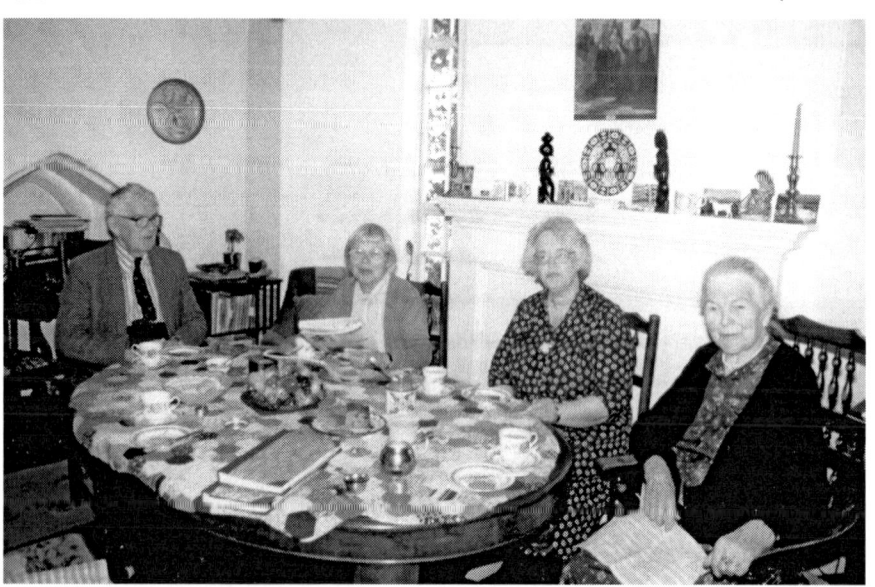

Father, Biddy Carrick, Benedicta and my Mother sharing a meal

was a good Green Line coach service passing the farm gate which enabled me to continue visits and enjoy some country air. I also saw Mother's elderly cousin Annie Mitchell at her home in north London. Several friends celebrated their 21st birthdays that autumn; I altered my bridesmaid's dress for the parties and usually took John. I was fond of him and we met most weekends.

Theoretical work was interesting but demanding with essays to be written each week. Handwriting was becoming difficult because of a cramp like pain, but it remained legible: I didn't want anything to interfere with my training. I much enjoyed working with patients and was pleased when the physically handicapped schoolchildren returned from holiday. These young patients had long term health problems and while working under supervision I learnt appropriate treatments. This experience was most useful later in my career when I worked with disabled children, first for Liverpool School Health Services and then at Alder Hey Hospital.

Our course was designed to give us experience in a variety of situations, including consultant outpatient clinics at the hospital, 'evening clinics' for patients who worked during the day, and visits to specialist units including chest and geriatric hospitals.

Father made regular visits to London for meetings and usually stayed with friends in Blackheath so we could meet. Problems arose over travel to Denmark Hill which I was finding more taxing: rail strikes and delays were frequent and with an increasing work load in the final year, I considered moving nearer the hospital. In addition there was great tension and strain at 17 Manor Way after the publication of the book *Honest to God* written by the Bishop. The Press waited outside the house and we had strict instructions not to speak to any lingering strangers. I spoke to Miss Olive Sands, whose brother had worked with Father as a fellow Archdeacon and lived near King's; she was a very well qualified and respected physiotherapist and, knowing the Robinsons agreed with a move, looked for accommodation for me. I answered advertisements for rooms near the hospital but nothing was suitable, though I had decided not to return to Manor Way after the Christmas holiday.

In the New Year 1962 I visited physiotherapy departments in Liverpool at The Royal, Walton (where there was a new department), and Alder Hey Children's hospitals as I planned to work in that area after qualifying the following December. Alder Hey was only five minute's bicycle ride from our house, but I was advised to gain general experience before specialising.

My future housing needs however were more immediate. Father suggested applying to Greyladies, a training college for women church workers situated in Lewisham. He had taken services at their chapel when we lived in Blackheath and knew there was extra accommodation for visitors. Although this would still involve public transport, the house was within easy walking distance of Lewisham station where I could take the direct line to King's. Shortly before returning to London I was relieved to hear that I had been accepted: a bedsitting room was available and breakfast and evening meals were provided during the week, with full board at weekends.

5
My Final Year

NINETEEN SIXTY-TWO STARTED with a very cold winter; trains were delayed and erratic so journeys to King's were difficult and I often arrived late. One day the trains were cancelled and I stopped a passing car and asked for a lift to Denmark Hill. Evening journeys were also difficult and I arrived back at Greyladies exhausted and cold; the staff were kind and made me welcome and my room was warm and comfortable but the journey was very taxing. Living in an institution was new for me and had advantages and disadvantages: Father could always stay at Greyladies when working in London, which was a bonus, but living in a close community of single women was trying at times. These two factors made me decide to enquire about accommodation nearer the hospital.

There were more 21st birthday parties, mostly in the Denmark Hill area. I didn't like late night travel back to Lewisham particularly in the winter, so missed many of these. My social life in Blackheath was full: playing squash at the Priory club, which was within cycling distance of Greyladies, enjoying meals with various friends and families including the Henkels, Robinsons and Canon Gordon Davies and family, and attending concerts at Goldsmiths College and the Festival Hall with John. I also saw Canon Sands and Olive, a member of the elite Hurlingham Club to which she invited me. Mrs Pichler with Mary and Peter, and Canon Reggie Houghton would appear from time to time to support me when I was missing my own family. When Elisabeth wrote telling me she was pregnant again I knitted more baby clothes as a change from embroidery which I was doing for relaxation; later she stayed in Eltham with Sarah, so we were able to meet. My parents and Petrena were most caring and gave me much moral support and encouragement, writing regularly and sending parcels of books and snacks.

I was again working at Thurlow Park School for handicapped children and we were preparing for the Intermediate exams in May. Some days I studied in the College library after our normal working day, making sure I was back at Greyladies in time for the evening meal. I had moved back to the wards in the spring when Miss Stewart suggested I see Dr Claydon, who looked after students at the physiotherapy school, as I had lost weight and was tense. I had bouts of diarrhoea that term and repeated sinus infections and nose bleeds, but being prone to the latter from early childhood, they didn't worry me. I also had some backache, not unusual for physiotherapists. Dr Claydon thought I was 'overwound' and prescribed tablets.

I was studying hard for the mock Intermediate exams, and met up with Gillian in Blackheath. We compared work, gave each other mock vivas and practised massage and other manual skills. Some evenings after work, college friends stayed late so we could revise together. I was happier in this last year at King's than I had been since my parents moved to Liverpool.

I went home for Easter and had a relaxing two weeks reading novels, gardening, shopping and walking in the countryside with the family. After the holiday Father and I travelled back to London; he had meetings and I was due to work with patients in the hydrotherapy pool. I still couldn't find suitable accommodation nearer the hospital so remained at Greyladies. We sat the two written exam papers early in the term, with a three-week interval before the practical. Unfortunately the latter was three days after my 21st birthday so I postponed celebrations till later. The practicals were again at Queen Square, and mine on a Friday; as we had the weekend free I went straight home to Liverpool to celebrate my birthday and end of exams with the family.

A Flat near to the Hospital

Margaret Jenkinson, a student friend in the set above me, had moved from a bed-sitting room in Herne Hill to a flat. Knowing I was looking for a room near the hospital she had shown me round. Although the accommodation was small and cooking facilities basic, it was within walking distance of the hospital, and after meeting Miss Southgate, the elderly owner, I accepted. Forty years on Margaret and I remain friends though we seldom meet, as she retired from physiotherapy to train for the priesthood and now has a Parish in the Carlisle Diocese.

Father knew the local vicar, Reverend Frank Bull at Herne Hill: he visited me and soon I was baby-sitting for his young family. I also became involved with residents at Atholl House, a Cheshire home in nearby Dulwich, helping with general domestic chores and befriending residents, my first contact with disabled adults in a home. Those who were able helped with domestic tasks, and some residents invited me to play table tennis. Many were wheelchair users and some also had limited arm movements, but I had to use my skill to give them a good game because of their expertise.

Living at Herne Hill, John and I saw more of each other, meeting up for games of tennis and squash; we were able to play on the hospital courts. We went to concerts at Goldsmiths College in New Cross, to dances and enjoyed meals out.

At the hospital I returned to the outpatient clinics; as finalists we were treating patients most of the day and had few lectures. A visit to Harefield Hospital for respiratory illnesses coincided with the annual Lord Mayor's Banquet for Bishops at the Mansion House where I was to accompany Father in Mother's place. I had to rush from Harefield to my lodging to change into evening dress, and then had the unforgettable thrill of walking up the steps of the Mansion

House with Father between the uniformed Guard of Honour. During the meal I had my first experience of a loving cup; fortunately my neighbour gave me instructions to turn, then bow my head to him before drinking, and repeating the ceremony to the next person; later, waiters brought each of us a finger bowl. I returned to my lodgings feeling elated.

Life was more relaxed, having finished intermediate exams and with the end of training in sight. Living at Herne Hill made socialising with fellow students easier and I was able to invite friends to tea, though kitchen facilities did not allow more substantial meals. We also played tennis and squash. One weekend I went to see mother's elderly cousin, Annie Mitchell, who lived in North Harrow; she gave me a beautiful ruby ring as a 21st birthday present. That summer was very hot and dry but life was good and fulfilling and my health was more stable.

Exam results were announced in late June: I was delighted to pass, but five of our set did not. We had mixed emotions: excitement that we would soon be qualified and responsible for the treatment of our own patients, earning money and independent, but sad to be leaving King's and our tutors. My rotation until the end of term was to the hydrotherapy pool, a placement I enjoyed, and would later find helpful for myself as a patient.

Summer Holidays

I RETURNED TO LIVERPOOL for the summer holiday and felt more familiar with the neighbourhood and family routine. Petrena was working by correspondence course towards membership of the Library Association and had also taken an exam. She was on holiday in North Wales, so I had a week at home with my parents before we went to Solva, near St David's. We stayed in a guesthouse overlooking the harbour, with wonderful views from our bedroom windows. We explored the beautiful countryside and coast, and Father and I enjoyed several swims in the sea despite chilly weather. Father patiently gave me driving lessons along the quiet roads.

On our return, I had an informal interview with Miss Leigh-Smith, Superintendent Physiotherapist at Walton General Hospital; she offered me a job subject to passing my finals. I stayed with Elisabeth at Stockton on Tees before returning to King's; she was expecting her second baby in September so was glad of help with Sarah.

Final Term

On return to King's I worked on the wards; as finalists we had just one lecture a day, spending the remaining time working with our own patients. For the lecture on treatment of patients who were being ventilated by 'the iron lung', I was nominated to be the model. It was a strange experience to be trapped in a box, though I could breathe myself, unlike patients who had to be ventilated to keep alive.

As my bed-sitter was not very comfortable I often stayed at the school in the evenings to study in the library. We were also able to attend part of The Chartered Society of Physiotherapy Annual Congress, and local branch meetings which were often more interesting.

We visited the Spinal Injury Unit at Stoke Mandeville. At Atholl House I was with patients who had been treated at the latter, and it was interesting to see the wards, equipment and therapy sessions for spinal injury patients. Roehampton Hospital, which specialised in artificial limbs (prostheses), was also interesting; seeing limbs being made as well as therapy rooms where patients first learnt to use their limbs was enlightening.

Miss Leigh-Smith had written from Liverpool asking for a reference. Miss Stewart said she would willingly give one but offered me a job on the staff at King's. I was naturally delighted, but thought I would probably move home to Liverpool.

My social life was full and when Petrena spent a weekend in London we stayed with friends in Blackheath. Elisabeth's second daughter was born in mid September, and I was delighted to be asked to be a godmother to Rachel Mary. John and I went to the Café Royal for his firm's dinner dance. Olive Sands again invited me to the Hurlingham Club where we enjoyed a walk in the grounds among the brilliantly coloured autumn leaves. Another weekend I stayed with my cousin Sue Hampson and her husband Bob in North London and had my first ride on a scooter. Living at Herne Hill I was able to see more of Bertram Simpson, former Bishop of Southwark, who lived there.

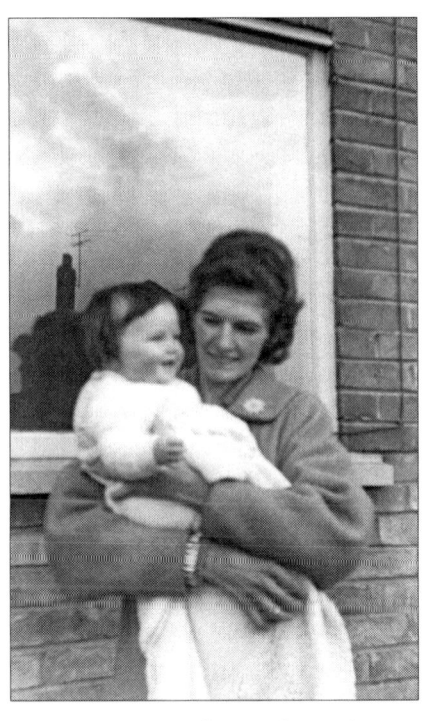

Jill holding her first God Daughter, Rachel Mary Ward-Lilley

Margaret Jenkinson, whose flat I had taken on, hadn't moved far and we played squash at the Medical School court, and also had meals together in her new flat. Pamela Welch, a school-friend, started nurse training at King's that autumn so we met from time to time.

I continued visits to Atholl House and enjoyed helping there. Having decided to move north after qualifying, I went sightseeing in London when I had free time and friends were busy: Westminster Abbey, St. Paul's Cathedral, Southwark Cathedral, the Houses of Parliament, the London Parks and some art galleries, including Dulwich Art Gallery which had some unexpected treasures for a small gallery, and the Imperial War Museum. Autumn was fine, sunny and mellow, and I was relieved to be able to walk or cycle through Ruskin Park to the hospital; I loved the freedom the bicycle gave me, similar to that I now experience when using my electric wheelchair.

At the end of September I saw Dr John Anderson, Consultant Physician at King's College Hospital, having been referred by Dr Claydon. Dr Anderson was also concerned about my weight and general condition and after a thorough examination and many blood tests, referred me to Miss Carden, a dietician, who prescribed 'Complan' a food supplement, the start of a long association. There weren't any fancy flavours in those days, but I found it palatable, and subsequently used it regularly for years. Unfortunately at the time we didn't know that I was sensitive to cow's milk, an ingredient of Complan. I was a patient of Dr Anderson, who was later Professor of Medicine at King's, until he retired 23 years later.

As my condition didn't improve, due it was thought to a weak immune system, I had to reduce practical work with patients to half the day at the beginning of November. Naturally I was concerned that I wouldn't get sufficient experience and practice before finals so I used the time to study in the school library. Eventually I was persuaded to go into hospital, while continuing my half day's practical work and attending any lectures. Thus I was introduced to Trundle ward, which I came to know very well over the years.

My work in the fracture clinic was not strenuous; at the time this was quite a new area for physiotherapists. We saw X-rays to check bone repair, and some patients were given immediate physiotherapy after removal of splints. One afternoon I went to a lecture on state registration for physiotherapists which had just been introduced. At weekends I was allowed to visit friends, do my usual chores, see to my correspondence, and attend chapel services, as long as I told the ward staff where I was going. I had nearly all my meals on the ward. Dr Anderson was worried not only about my immune system and weight loss, but also about metabolism and absorption. At first I was in a single room and received treatment during the evenings and overnight. A Ryle's tube was inserted via my nose into my stomach, through which various 'concoctions' were dripped. I soon became used to the routine and discomfort, though after the first treatment I had uncontrollable diarrhoea, so the fluids were adjusted and that solved the problem.

Final exams were on 21st November 1962 at Queen Square. Fortunately the number 68 bus passed King's and went within five minutes walk of the Square. The exam consisted of practical treatments on student 'guinea pigs' with various conditions; we were observed and questioned as we treated them. A week later a fellow student, Fay, came to the ward to tell me I had passed. Those of us who qualified left King's officially on the day results came through. We agreed to keep in touch with one another and most of us have done so, meeting for reunions at varying intervals. I remained in Trundle ward, confined to bed with constant medication. After a week I was allowed up but had a setback before gradually improving.

The exact cause of my illness and diagnosis were not known. I had worked hard, both physically and mentally but that didn't account for the troublesome diarrhoea and other symptoms, but eventually I made a good recovery, which we hoped was complete. While in hospital I heard that I had been accepted as a junior physiotherapist at Walton Hospital starting in January 1963, and was told that I could go home to Liverpool for Christmas.

One of the nurses told me she had a scooter for sale, which I recklessly bought for £35. She agreed to ride it to Euston station for me to take to Liverpool; I wished I had asked her how to unlock the steering, and had a worrying few minutes until a porter solved that problem.

Before leaving I visited the School of Physiotherapy to thank Miss Evelyn Stewart and her staff for their tuition and understanding during my three years of training. She was a wonderful Principal and great support throughout my training and when I was ill. It is thanks to her that I completed my training and came through my illness, and subsequently qualified as a physiotherapist. She has kept in touch since then and we have met on two or three occasions. She set a great example to us all.

6

To Work in Liverpool

Returning to Liverpool for Christmas 1962 there were just ten days to buy gifts for the family and friends and help with preparations. Elisabeth and family were to join us; Petrena had already helped make the Christmas puddings and decorate the cake.

I had certain formalities to complete before starting work at Walton in the New Year: joining the local bank and insuring the scooter. My parents suggested I try riding the scooter around the extensive grounds of our house before going out on the road. Father offered to give me driving lessons, hoping I would sell the scooter and learn to drive a car; I bought a driving licence.

Christmas was jolly and we all went to the Cathedral carols, which were a wonderful start to the celebrations. The vast Cathedral, though still not completed, had a very special staccato sound which echoed round the building. It was always a thrill to see Father in procession at special services or when he was invited to officiate. The Dean (or Provost depending on its origin) is in charge of the administration and he (or she) may invite the Bishop to celebrate or preach apart from Christmas Day,

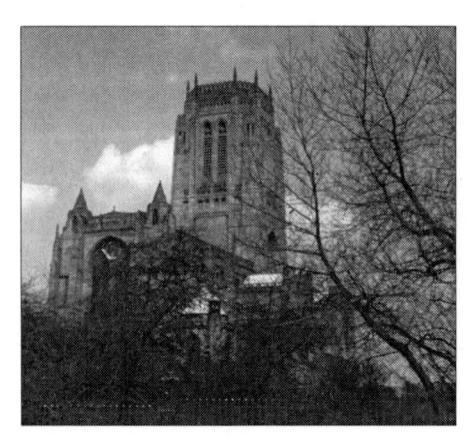

Liverpool Cathedral

※ To Work in Liverpool ※

Easter Sunday and Pentecost Sunday when he has the right to take part in the services. Ernie Clark, a parish priest in a nearby suburb of Liverpool, joined us for Christmas tea. He had worked with Father at the South London Church Fund and had no relatives.

As parishioners and members of St Mary's Church in West Derby we joined in the post Christmas party at the Parish hall. My father's predecessor had been the Vicar as well as Bishop of Warrington and although Father had not taken on the parish, we had strong links with St Mary's.

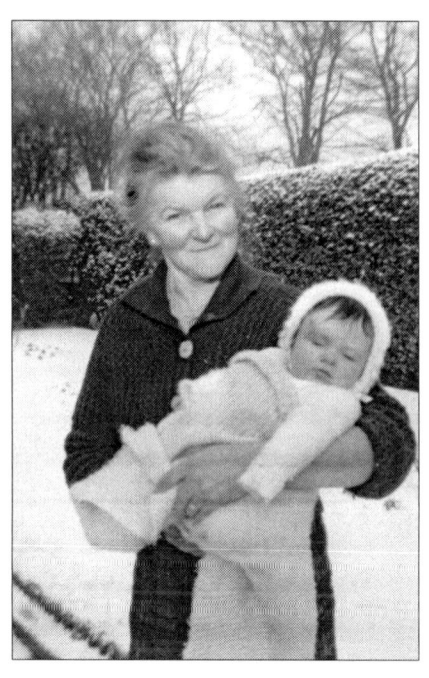

Mother holding Rachel when they visited at the "White Christmas"

The winter of 1963 was severe with heavy falls of snow and ice, which Liverpool usually escapes because of salt in the atmosphere from the sea. The snow froze and transport was difficult. Elisabeth and Brian had to extend their stay as the roads over the Pennines were impassable, but we enjoyed the longer visit and the children loved playing in the snow. I wanted to practise riding my scooter to enable me to get to work, but that was impossible as the driveway and side roads were frozen for three months. However our vast garage proved just big enough to be my first trial area.

There was a large correspondence to attend to after the excitements of Christmas, having received many cards and letters from friends at the hospital, and Father's friends who had supported me so much during the time I was homesick and later ill. I also wanted to write to Dr Anderson and Miss Stewart, not being sure I had thanked them and my friends enough for all the help and encouragement they had given me.

Physiotherapist at Walton Hospital

I FOUND A BIG change from working as a student in the busy departments at King's to being a member of staff in a new hospital. At first there were very few patients in the out-patients department, but that soon changed and after a week there was an evening clinic; that was a very long day. I knew something of the Liverpool dialect but still needed to ask Annie Cropper, our homehelp, for interpretations.

Fortunately our house was a short walk from a bus to the hospital in Queen's Drive, the ring road; sometimes Father would give me a lift. When the weather improved and with more confidence riding the scooter on quiet roads near our home, I tried riding to work, but felt insecure and soon realised that a scooter was not my ideal choice of vehicle. After a couple of months I sold it, had professional driving lessons, and saved to buy a car.

The variety of work in outpatients was enjoyable and every day was different. At lunch times there was a very active 'bridge group', but not being an ardent card player I preferred to read. Sometimes I felt the department head disapproved of my not joining in: she was very keen on the game. Departmental outings to the ice skating rink were also not a success; I preferred warmer sports like tennis, squash, table tennis and badminton. Although I got on well with most of the staff, there was a feeling that being a southerner and also the daughter of a bishop, I was somehow different. One rather 'stuffy' member of staff thought that clergymen were very strict and puritanical, ruling over their households and daughters

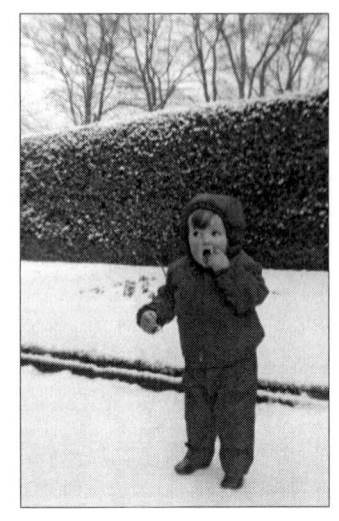

Sarah in the snow at St Martin's

with a rod of iron. I teased her by saying that after one staff outing, which had ended rather later than expected, Father waited behind the front door and beat me. She believed me in spite of reassurances that my father was a wonderful, caring person and most approachable and would never do anything like that.

Friends and Leisure Activities

I MADE GOOD FRIENDS in Liverpool including some from work; Jean Thompson, a senior physiotherapist introduced me to the English Speaking Union, whose meetings were enjoyable at first, but after six months I needed something more practical and enrolled for typing and pottery evening classes. I explored Chester and the Wirral with new friends from work, and went to the theatre and shopping outings. A colleague, Alvon Sausman, also lived in West Derby, and later we corresponded about our Assistance dogs: she had a Guide Dog for the Blind and I have a Dog for the Disabled. Alvon has since died. Ann Davies (née Borrows) and I, both newly qualified, started work at Walton the same day. We became good friends and I went to Ann and Barry's wedding in Liverpool. When they moved to Barnack, near Stamford, they invited me to stay several times and we had great fun playing with their two children, Richard and Rachel, on the ancient site known as 'hills and holes' near their home. Carole Dennis and I met through our parents; her father was vicar in Bootle. She worked as a secretary in Liverpool and we met for coffee and shopping in the city centre until our ways parted.

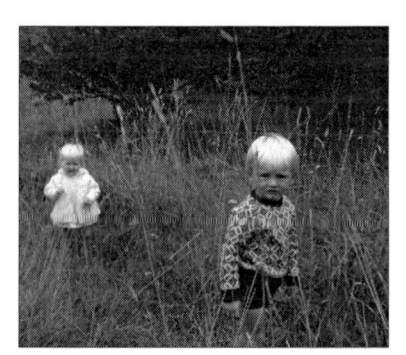

Richard and Rachel at "The hills and the holes" Barnack

I became involved with the Girl Guide movement again and was

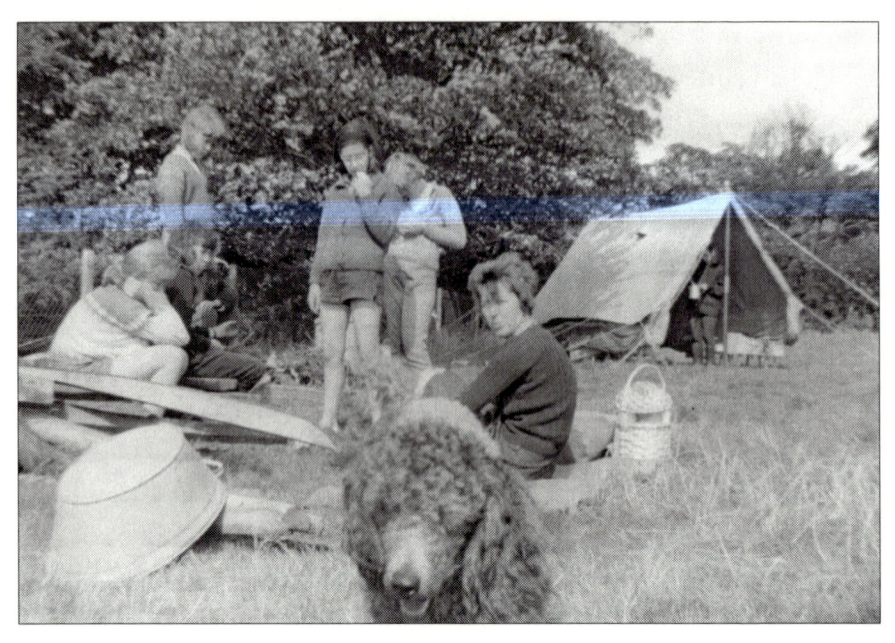

At Guide camp

assistant at the West Derby company, enjoying the weekly meetings, taking charge in Captain's absence, and being appointed assessor for some proficiency badges. In spring and summer we practised making campfires for cooking, erected tents, identified trees and plants, and went on outings in preparation for summer camps. Sometimes the guides would come to the 'den' they had made in our large garden for relaxation and fun.

In the winter months Petrena and I enjoyed many games of table tennis, sometimes with friends, on a full size table at home. I had become quite skilful since playing regularly with residents at Atholl House. We had certain responsibilities with the running of the house, including cleaning and preparation of meals. We tried Scottish Dancing in the village hall but I didn't enjoy it; Mother said, 'I was all arms and legs'. Knitting was another activity, stimulated by Elisabeth's two girls who were growing rapidly and needing new sweaters. It was good having a wage again but I was careful with spending so as to save money.

In spring I started professional driving lessons; Father continued to take me for driving practice initially on quiet roads, then he began to meet me at work to give me experience of driving home on the busy ring road. Later I drove him to some of his church duties further afield.

Visitors and Visiting

Auntie Florrie and Uncle Bob came to stay; they were a gentle couple and Mother's closest relations. I visited my cousin Judy and her husband Ian at their home in Staffordshire. We had lost touch since childhood and now we were living nearer it was a good opportunity to get to know them.

Early in the summer I had a bad attack of shingles, affecting the area around the right side of my ribs; my GP gave me injections to relieve the pain. As a result my general health deteriorated and Miss Leigh-Smith thought that it would be wise to see a specialist. Dr Honey at Rodney Street, where many doctors had their private rooms, much to my relief gave me the all clear, and reassured me that my health was reasonable for a person of my slender build after a bad attack of shingles.

The summer weather was mixed that year but Mother was fortunate to have a fine day for her first garden party in Liverpool which raised £29 for charity; a reasonable sum for the time.

We were members of the church tennis club and played with other members or practised with family and friends. Petrena had taken on the task of delivering parish magazines to a high rise block of flats and I joined her in climbing the endless flights of stairs. Whenever the opportunity arose I went to the country for a walk with friends or to see a stately home. I was certainly enjoying life and making the most of my leisure time.

Holiday

IN LATE SUMMER James and Joyce Rogers, Uncle Roland's sister and brother in law, invited me for a ten day visit to their home in Dumfries. He was a consultant psychiatrist at the Crichton Royal Hospital, very near their home, and Joyce a trained nurse, busy bringing up their four young children. My parents drove me to Keswick for a coach to Dumfries. I explored the area both on my own and with the family, who lived within walking distance of the town. The museum contained memorabilia of Robert Burns whose statue was in the town centre. I went by coach to Kirkcudbright and Rockliffe, and enjoyed the chance to eat fresh salmon. I cycled to Kingsholm quay, Ladyfield, Kippford and around the colourful gardens surrounding the Crichton Royal Hospital. James let me drive their eight gear Landrover; good practice for my driving test in a few weeks. Joyce was a keen tennis player and we had lively games at the hospital courts. It was also blackberrying time so I helped the family stock up with the free succulent fruits. The days passed quickly. The return coach journey through the Lake District and Lancashire, though slow, was interesting and added to my geographical knowledge.

Home Life and Work

A WEEK LATER I took the driving test and failed; disappointed I resolved to get more practice and retake as soon as possible. I so wanted to drive myself to work and take Mother out. Father nobly gave me even more opportunities to drive our car, both in built up areas and the country; Liverpool Diocese is large and Father's work involved travelling to any parish in the area, so I became his chauffeuse whenever I could. I also had regular lessons to prepare for my re-take. Typing and pottery courses continued at the local night school and several friends from the physiotherapy department joined me at the pottery class; we all enjoyed 'messing about with clay'. I wasn't artistic but enjoyed the soft feel of clay and still have some of my attempts at pottery from this time, and from later years when we lived in Birmingham and I attended a class at Cannon Hill Park Art Centre with an occupational therapist.

Evening clinics at work were always rushed, though the days were more relaxed with fewer patients. One evening we had a 'work's outing' to Clatterbridge Hospital, over the river Mersey, and it was interesting to meet other local physiotherapists and see their department. There were several foreign physiotherapists from Germany, Holland and Scandinavia on the staff, and they seemed pleased to come to a family home, as they were in lodgings. Our house in Sandfield Park was large enough for all the family to lead fairly independent lives, when we wanted to. When my friends came to the house I could prepare a meal and entertain them without intruding on my parents, though if they were home, they were always pleased to meet friends.

The note to renew my subscription to The Chartered Society of Physiotherapy reminded me I had been qualified and working for twelve months. There were no doubts about my chosen career: I enjoyed working in a general hospital putting knowledge learnt during training into practice, but looked forward to an opportunity to work with children. This was also my first year of living full time in Liverpool; I had made good friends at work and socially, and was happy living at home again.

My parents were always busy and Father had various commitments in London and at York where members of the northern dioceses met for Synod (meetings of the clergy and laity); Mother sometimes went with him, leaving Auntie Margaret, Petrena and me in charge of the house and dog walking.

Christmas 1963 was quiet, with Auntie Florrie staying with us; sadly her husband had died of a sudden heart attack. On Boxing Day we enjoyed our usual family walk on the shore at Formby, looking for red squirrels which can be seen there. Petrena and I entertained some of our friends and I joined some of the socialising at the hospital; many wards and departments had open house with drinks and nibbles; it was good to meet colleagues informally.

My New Year's resolution was to learn dressmaking: we wore uniform at work, but I needed more formal clothes for official events with my parents, so I borrowed Mother's old treadle machine, which though basic was reliable. I was glad to have help from Auntie Margaret who was a good dressmaker and had made dresses and skirts for me in the past, but experienced a sense of achievement when my first outfit was completed; I continued to make most of my own clothes for many years.

The Head of Department was still worried about my health and weight and wanted me to see one of the hospital doctors for a check up. My GP thought it unnecessary and we were both annoyed when she insisted on the medical; again I was passed as fit for work.

During the spring of 1964 I had several short holidays: first to

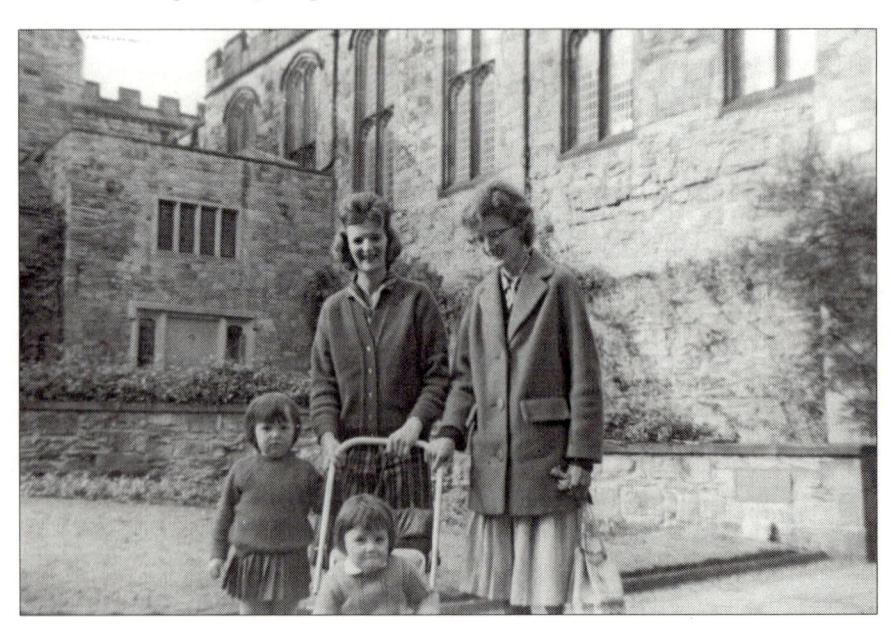

Elisabeth pushing Rachel with Sarah and Jill in Durham

stay with Elisabeth and family at their home in Stockton on Tees when I enjoyed helping to look after my goddaughter, Rachel; then, with Father, shared driving to London, via Cambridge. Father had engagements in Cambridge so I stayed with Prue Murphy, née Green, a school friend who lived at nearby Royston; we chatted for hours about physiotherapy and nursing (she had trained as a nurse at Barts). Then Father and I went to London where he had meetings. I stayed with Gladys Pichler at Brand's Hatch, visiting more school and physiotherapy friends, including Pat Lisle (née Dee) who had married Chris and moved to Orpington since qualifying. Tragically Pat died in March 2010, a few months after our 50th reunion.

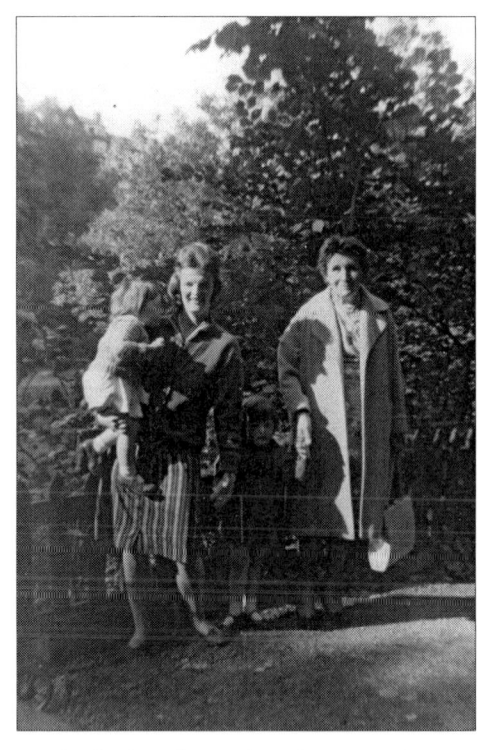

Elisabeth with Sarah and Auntie Florrie

A few weeks later Father led a party of pilgrims, including the Stroud family from Salisbury, to the Holy Land. The evenings were free and finding they shared common interests, the Strouds and Father spent time together resulting in a friendship which has continued to the present day. The Strouds had a lakeside cottage, Swan Lake, near Shaftesbury and invited Father to use it; subsequently we had many happy holidays there, and as a result decided to find a house in the Salisbury area when Father retired in 1977. More of that later.

In May I passed my driving test and became second chauffeuse for the family when I could borrow Father's car, as neither Mother, Auntie nor Petrena drove. Buying my own car was a priority as I

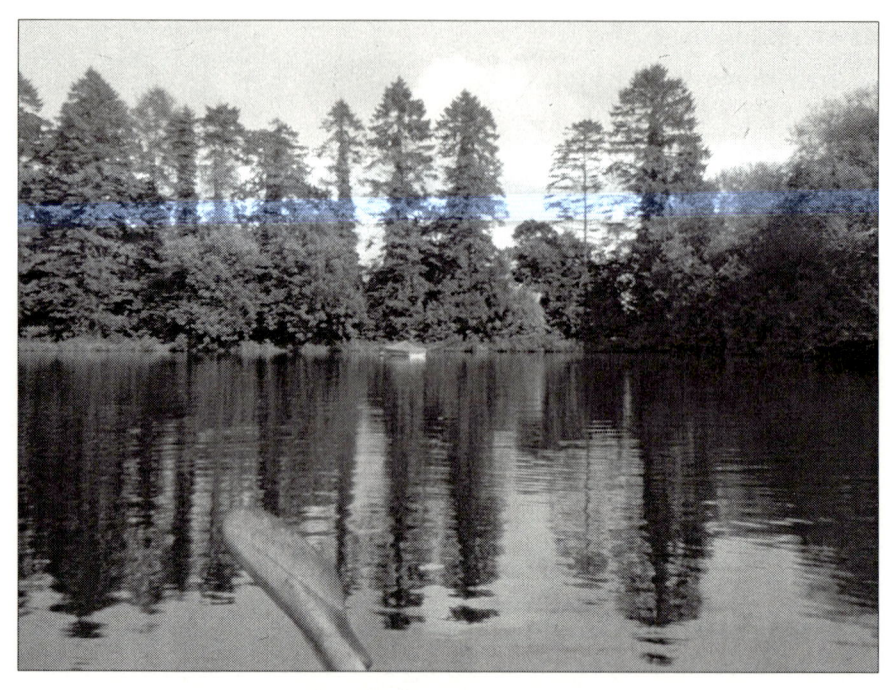

The lake at Swanlake Cottage

wanted to explore the Wirral, Lake District, Keswick and parts of north Wales with Petrena and friends. Father found a second hand Mini, which seemed a good buy at the time and I was delighted, till it kept breaking down. A mechanic who Father knew and trusted checked the car and detected the mileage clock had been turned back; within a month the garage refunded my money under guarantee.

I was very disappointed, as I liked the car, but that experience put me off Minis. Before long I found a maroon Anglia which lasted for several years. Proudly I drove to Guide camp, held at Standish, north of Liverpool, for the Whitsun holiday and had my first experience of camping as a Guider; I enjoyed it, despite being woken in the night by guides, sick after their midnight feast. Elisabeth and family had a summer holiday in Deganwy, North Wales and I drove off to visit them, thoroughly enjoying time spent with my nieces on the beach there.

✳ *To Work in Liverpool* ✳

Moving House

During the late summer my parents started house hunting; after weeks of searching they found a 'gem' in Great Crosby. This was a good location from a Diocesan point of view, as the Bishop of Liverpool lived in a suburb on the east of Liverpool and Great Crosby was on the west, with Church House, the office and the Cathedral in the centre. The new house called 'Cupplesfield' was a reasonable size, attractive and had a manageable, well laid out and maintained garden. It seemed an excellent investment for the Diocese. My parents were given the go-ahead to move in Spring 1965. We were delighted for none of us liked St Martin's, and the dampness had certainly adversely affected my health and contributed to back and leg pains as well as constant colds. As the time for the move approached, we had work to do at Cupplesfield and most weekends I drove Mother, Auntie Margaret and Petrena to Crosby with our mops and buckets. We

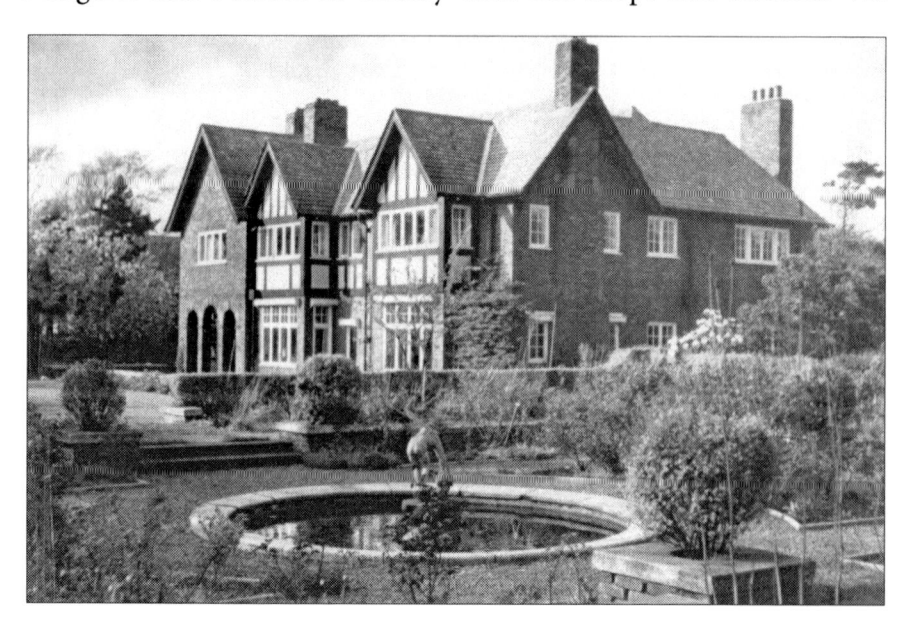

View of Cupplesfield from the back garden

measured for curtains and carpets, scrubbed floors and cupboards when the workmen finished the decorating, and when the weather permitted Petrena and Auntie tackled the garden, which though well laid out, needed tidying. During the week we tidied cupboards and packed at Sandfield Park; fortunately we hadn't accumulated too much since our move from London.

Paediatric Physiotherapist

In August an advertisement appeared for a paediatric physiotherapist to work for Liverpool City Council, and after interview and medical, I was offered the job starting in October. I gave in my notice at Walton, happy that at last my dream of working with children was to come true. The superintendent physiotherapist of school health, Mrs Bridges, introduced me to Greenbank School near Sefton Park, where the atmosphere was happy and relaxed, and I met some of the children. They were aged between 5 and 16 and had various disabilities, including spina bifida, cerebral palsy and muscular dystrophy. I had already treated disabled children during my student placements at schools in Tulse Hill, the children's wards at King's and at Belgrave Hospital, the small outpatient unit nearby.

Shortly after this, I had my first private patient: Jean Thompson, a colleague at Walton hospital, asked me to continue treating a woman who lived near my home. This was the beginning of a long friendship, both professional and later personal, with Miss Dorothy Stewart, a gentle person from whom I learnt a great deal over the years, as well as trying to help her. Although we moved to Crosby, ten miles to the west, a few months later, I was able to visit her by car, and continued seeing her for six years.

After leaving Walton Hospital on 24th September 1964, and with ten days holiday owing, I took Auntie Florrie to see Elisabeth and her family at Stockton on Tees. We enjoyed exploring County

Durham; the hill top position of the city of Durham and Cathedral was most impressive, with views of spacious moors. Mother was admitted to Broad Green Hospital for a planned operation the day after our return. Auntie Florrie, who was very close to her, stayed with us so she could visit and keep her company when she was discharged home. I prepared to start my new job with children – my long term professional aim.

A Short Interval Working for School Health

I REPORTED TO GREENBANK School on October 5th to start work with the superintendent physiotherapist. First I had to learn the school routine: being Roman Catholic, the children had Confessions one morning each week, so there was no physiotherapy till midday, and another morning we took the children swimming. It was a challenge encouraging some of them into the water, but rewarding to see them laughing and splashing around with their friends after a few sessions. My work was varied and interesting, each child needing help with their specific problems.

After a week Mrs Bridges left me to treat the children on my own. This was a change from the large number of staff at Walton, but I got on with work, organising my timetable and liaising with teachers, advising them on positioning for the children and gaining feedback from them.

The school was opposite Sefton Park, one of the chain of attractive parks around Liverpool and during the lunch break I enjoyed some fresh air strolling there, watching the changing season.

After a few weeks I was invited to attend out of school events and outings, for instance, swimming galas, plays, and one day Chester Zoo. The children were pleased to have support from teachers, helpers and physiotherapist, a good example of holistic medicine, though we didn't call it that.

I also had to treat children at various school clinics around the city, some of whom regarded their treatment as fun time off school. Many had flat feet or poor posture, which could be remedied by exercise. Following a course of successful treatment they were sent back to the referring doctor. To my surprise and disappointment, several returned. Since there was no system of direct communication between doctor and physiotherapist, the children had to be relied on to demonstrate their improvement to the doctor. I thought the latter didn't consider my treatment successful and was perplexed until one young lad confessed they enjoyed coming to the clinic and missing school, so they adopted their former bad posture or flat feet in order to be sent back for more physiotherapy.

Eventually I set up a system of mailing written reports to the doctors, because these children, often from poor homes, needed all the education they could get. Occasionally I attended clinics at the special schools, one immediately next to our home in Sandfield Park, discussing with medical and school staff the general well-being of the children and giving advice about seating and posture. This was not very satisfactory as I was unable to see the children regularly.

An advantage of working for school health was no weekend duties, nor evening clinics. In the autumn I enrolled for a motor maintenance class: I thought I should learn what was under the bonnet of my car. Most of the students were expert mechanics but at least I learnt how to check batteries and tyres. As there wasn't a squash club nearby I joined a Badminton Club at St James' Church in West Derby. Many of us had to play table tennis, as there was only one badminton court. Guides took up at least one or two evenings a week so I was hardly at home: the joy of being in my twenties and full of youthful energy.

I visited Miss Stewart on my way home from work each week. She had severe rheumatoid arthritis, among other things, and was brave and uncomplaining, living with her younger sister, Edna, who taught at a Liverpool school. I treated her deformed, swollen joints and did as much as possible to relieve the pain and maintain mobility.

Her oldest sister suffered from the same disease, but her condition was so severe she could no longer be cared for at home and was in a nursing home near the centre of Liverpool; occasionally I visited her, taking parcels between the two sisters. Later my Miss Stewart had to go into the same nursing home, a sad move, for her older sister had died there. Before this she sometimes went to Parkhouse nursing home in Crosby for respite care, and as they had no regular physiotherapist, she asked me to continue treating her there. Later when we moved south I visited her whenever we returned to Liverpool.

When Edna wrote to tell me of her death I felt the loss, for she had become a fine example of a person in great pain and distress who lived her life graciously, complaining little. Edna sent me her small tablet boxes which are treasured as a memento of my friend and patient.

At home we entertained family and friends as well as visiting clergymen from abroad, among them was the Bishop of the Arctic, who came to Liverpool for meetings. Mother was in demand to open parish Christmas Fayres, and as Father was often doing similar tasks elsewhere I acted as chauffeuse. Membership of our guide company had grown over the year, giving more work for the volunteers; I was working to complete the Guide Warrant course.

When school and clinics broke up for the Christmas holidays, I was sent to work at Alder Hey Children's Hospital, a five minute bicycle ride from our house. This was work I really enjoyed and wanted to do, so when Mr Ruben, the head physiotherapist, offered me a permanent job, the opportunity was too good to miss.

We went to Norton to spend Christmas with Elisabeth, Brian and their family. Elisabeth was again pregnant and glad of any help, and we had a family orientated Boxing Day with friends of hers who also had a young family. The north east was icey cold with snow and we were relieved to find Liverpool milder.

In the New Year I continued at Alder Hey until the school clinics at Bootle, Walton and Dingle re-opened, when my day was divided between the two. When the children returned to Greenbank School I joined them. Treating them was fulfilling and the co-operation of the teaching staff excellent, but I felt professionally isolated and rarely saw Mrs Bridges. Communication about clinic patients hadn't improved noticeably despite my efforts.

Soon after returning to Greenbank I had my first experience of tutoring a student in paediatric physiotherapy. With no training in supervision I had to think back to my own student days. The challenge was stimulating, thought provoking, and good training for later in my career at Birmingham Children's Hospital, when I regularly tutored students. Mrs Bridges was unwell and off work so it was good to have a student's company which helped overcome the feeling of isolation.

In mid February 1965 my nephew, James Alexander Ward Lilley was born and Mother went to Norton to help Elisabeth. Petrena had a break before taking more library association exams, so Auntie Margaret and I kept house for Father and Judy. My application for the post at Alder Hey Hospital was accepted from the beginning of March so I gave up working for school health but promised to keep in touch.

7
To Alder Hey and the Best of my Working Days as a Physiotherapist ~ 1965-68

Spring 1965 was certainly a time of change: I started work at Alder Hey Children's Hospital, West Derby on 1st March and we moved house to Great Crosby on 5th April. It was ironic that Alder Hey was a five-minute bike ride from our previous house in Sandfield Park, West Derby but twelve miles from Cupplesfield in Great Crosby. However both the new job and new home were worth the effort of the longer journey.

Work

Having said 'farewell' to my young patients and staff at Greenbank School and the clinics with some sadness, I looked forward to a permanent post at Alder Hey. It was the main children's hospital in the area, as well as having the regional burns unit. A separate children's hospital in Myrtle Street looked after new-born babies; if specialist facilities were needed, sick babies were transferred to Alder Hey.

We were a staff of five physiotherapists at Alder Hey including the superintendent, Mr Rubin, plus an excellent orderly, who looked after us as well as assisting with patients. At first my work was part time in the main outpatients department and part time on medical wards, each member of staff being responsible for physiotherapy on certain wards. Later I took on treating children with cerebral palsy at a separate wooden building then called the Spastics Centre, five minutes walk from the main department.

On the wards we were always busy treating chest conditions including bronchiolitis, cystic fibrosis, pneumonia and bronchiectasis, as well as surgical, orthopaedic and burns patients. In addition children with heart conditions, muscle weakness or other chronic diseases often succumbed to breathing problems in the winter.

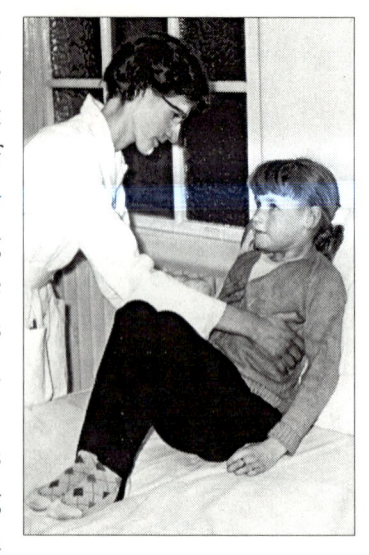

Acutely ill children were treated in isolation wards, where we worked closely with the staff. Chest treatments in particular had to be fitted in with feeding times, for the babies were very ill and needed frequent small meals. We gently percussed and vibrated the chest wall to loosen sputum and assist the child to cough. Percussion was performed by patting the chest wall with cupped hands, the pressure used depending on the size and condition of the child. For tiny babies we used our fingertips. The child was placed in the appropriate position to help drain fluid from a lung or part of a lung, especially if there were signs of collapse or a build up of fluid or sputum. If the sputum was tenacious a steam tent was helpful, and when necessary with very small babies or those children who couldn't cough, we used suction. This was done aseptically by inserting a special catheter attached to a suction machine into the breathing tubes via the nose, and clearing the mouth at the same time.

Most responded well, but before they went home, parents were taught how to percuss the chest and positioning for postural draining

✳ To Alder Hey ✳

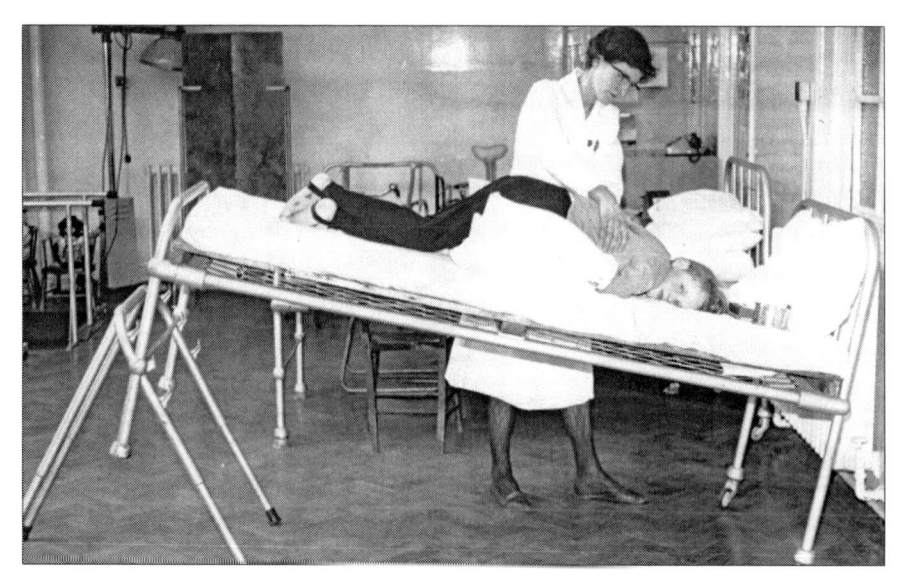

Jill in the Outpatients Department at Alder Hey Hospital treating a patient with chest problems: (opposite page) with deep breathing and chest vibrations (above) by Postural drainage with breathing exercises and percussion

to prevent recurrence of infection; children with cystic fibrosis would require this regimen for the rest of their lives.

Dr Robert Todd, a chest consultant, corresponded with me until his recent death; he was a great man. However, I still correspond with Mrs Bronwen Hughes (née Jones) an occupational therapist at the Spastics Centre, with whom I worked. Bronwen lived in Southport just north of Crosby; we became friendly and met up at weekends or after work. Later in January 1968 when Bronwen married Dr John Hughes, a GP, she invited me to attend both the wedding and reception. I was pleased she continued to work after she married, as we had developed a relaxed and successful method of working together. Other friends were Jean Maguire, a dental assistant who also lived in Crosby so shared my transport, and Dorothy Ross, a ward sister on one of the surgical wards. Her brother was ordained as a minister, giving us a common interest; sadly both have since died. During staff holidays I usually treated patients on her ward, and became friendly with a young lad, A, who had a serious bowel disorder and required repeated admission.

The parents of a baby whom I treated from a few months old until he was discharged completely well aged 2, also send me a card every Christmas and in 1997 visited me in Salisbury with their fit and healthy son.

Soon after I started work Mr Rubin, the superintendent, arranged a morning's instruction at Myrtle Street, in the treatment of clubfoot by manipulation followed by specific physiotherapy. This involved gently manipulating the foot, encouraging corrective active movement by stroking the foot with cotton wool, and then strapping or splinting the foot in the corrected position.

Treating children in general outpatients and on the wards, with three afternoons a week specialising in the treatment of children with cerebral palsy, proved an interesting caseload. Dr Derham, in charge of the Spastics Centre, also requested I sometimes attend his other clinics to discuss whether physiotherapy could benefit a patient.

Cerebral Palsy

The Spastics Centre was housed in a rickety wooden building with a high ceiling and an incomplete partition between the physiotherapy and occupational therapy rooms, where two full time occupational therapists worked. There was a small office run by a lively secretary, Renée, a doctor's consulting room, staff and storerooms, with a corridor for equipment. Jean, the orderly, turned her hand to whatever needed doing, from cleaning the floor to toileting the children, or helping with positioning of a child, an important part of therapy for children with cerebral palsy.

Cerebral palsy is caused by damage to the brain at or near the time of birth and there are numerous causes and manifestations. We liked to have these patients when first diagnosed, ideally as babies, and found early treatment gave better results, but some children were not referred till later. Several methods of physiotherapy were practised at that time; I followed one which encouraged and trained normal patterns of development from babyhood onwards and discouraged abnormal patterns and postures. Every child was different and treatment progressed according to the individual.

The staff worked together as a team: if there was a particular challenge such as head control, sitting-balance, standing, or using a limb the occupational therapist would use reinforcing play activities. For example, if a child had difficulty using one hand or arm the physiotherapist would try to retrain normal patterns of movement while reducing any muscle spasm and unwanted movements, while the occupational therapist would encourage play activities with toys needing two hands to operate. Likewise if there was a problem with control of the head position, I would place the child on its tummy and encourage him or her to lift the head, attracting their attention by playing with a toy. Most children with cerebral palsy required long term treatment with regular reviews, and parents were shown exercises to do with their children every day.

Spina Bifida

We also treated children with spina bifida, which seemed more prevalent in those days. Perhaps this is because a link has been found between folic acid deficiency and its incidence, so that fewer babies are born with the condition now because mothers are given folic acid during pregnancy.

The condition arises when the fetal spinal cord doesn't develop fully, leaving a gap in the bones which should enclose the cord, and exposing the spinal nerves to damage. This results in varying degrees of muscle weakness or paralysis and lack of sensation in the back and legs, and sometimes lack of control of bladder and bowels, depending on the level of damage to the spinal cord. Some patients also suffer from hydrocephalus when the fluid surrounding the brain doesn't drain properly, leading to possible brain damage and an enlarged skull. An operation to close the gap in the bony spinal column is essential as early as possible to prevent infection and further damage to the nerves. Surgery can also be carried out to insert a drain to reduce pressure on the brain and skull. Physiotherapy aims to help normal development and mobility and prevent muscle contractions; walking aids may be needed.

Burns

Work in the burns unit was sometimes stressful. The children suffered extreme pain, especially in the early stages, and we weren't the most popular people, because we needed to encourage maintenance of joint movement and muscle strength as soon as possible. When children are acutely ill they don't want strangers doing anything to them, but once over the acute stage they usually recover quickly. (By contrast, progress with children with cerebral palsy is usually slow, but equally rewarding when even a little progress is made.) When children who had suffered burns were on their way to recovery, life became more fun for both them and therapists, as we helped mobilise their bodies and get them walking, preparing for life at home. Once children started to recover, pain and problems were forgotten and they were eager to return to playing and having fun.

Patients suffering from burns or scalds were usually in hospital for long periods and we became involved in their lives as well as with their families. Often they had to return for more cosmetic or plastic surgery and it was good to see how they were coping with their lives again. The work was interesting: having read a recent paper suggesting that ultrasound might relieve scar tissue, I researched the possibility of applying this to the treatment of young children. While Pauline Scott, the electrotherapy lecturer at King's was supportive, the consultant of the burns unit suggested we should wait for further evidence of benefit.

Case Histories

J, A DELIGHTFUL child aged 6, came from a distance with her parents or grandparents. She had cerebral palsy with severe spasms in her legs, and her family were so keen to help that they installed parallel bars the length of their garden so she could play outdoors with her friends. We worked hard to improve her mobility and she made good progress, and we transferred care to her local school health.

G, an adorable five-year-old from Australia, with curly auburn hair and a mischievous smile, had cerebral palsy; he enjoyed the fresh air and when possible we moved the parallel bars on to the grass outside the department for his walking practice. Having had several operations on his legs, we spent a lot of time trying to help him walk and he made some progress before moving to another area, when we lost touch.

B, aged two, was another severely disabled young boy with cerebral palsy, who had very limited communication; understandably he became frustrated when he could not let us know what he wanted. His parents were dedicated to helping him and brought him for treatment regularly and I adapted his exercises, which his parents did at home, as he developed. The communication aids now available were sadly only ideas at that time, as many of my young patients' lives would have been greatly improved by such equipment. Bradley died young, by which time his parents had a healthy girl which must have been some compensation.

No-one would forget seven year old E, who had Down's syndrome, because of her constant repetitive talking. Down's syndrome is a genetic disease, which manifests itself by mental retardation, and possibly some physical disorders. The occupational therapists treated her but she greeted everyone she saw.

A long-term patient was a teenager who had tragically become paralysed from the waist downwards as the result of a spinal tumour. He made good progress, eventually learning to walk short distances with crutches, using a wheelchair for longer outings. He was a keen model maker and during his long stay made me one of his model ships; sadly, it fell to pieces during one of our house moves.

Another rewarding patient was a young lad of four, acutely ill with Guillain Barré syndrome who was completely paralysed from the neck down.

This illness, thought to be viral, causes spreading paralysis of nerves, nerve roots, spinal cord, brain and meninges separately or combined. It is a frightening condition but usually reversible. At first he needed ventilation and I treated his chest using percussion and suction to clear the secretions, while also performing passive movements of his limbs to maintain the range of movement in the joints and muscles. Thankfully he made an excellent recovery and after a few weeks l was breathlessly chasing him on his tricycle up and down the hospital corridors.

Early in 1967 I became involved with a child who was one of twins; the girl was healthy and well but the boy, M, had cerebral palsy. He was very alert but could not communicate by speech or signing, though his facial expressions were indicative of thoughts. M was very attractive with a mass of curly hair. The parents requested that I treat him privately at home; parents, grandparents, other relatives and friends were all involved. Treatment and correct posture, supported by pillows, had to be part of their way of life in twenty four-hour care. Doctors and therapist had to support the family and help them accept the condition and its unfavourable prognosis. I treated ML for the next three years until we moved house, and during that time he made great progress with his head control, sitting balance and mobility, much to his obvious delight.

During the summer we gained an additional member of staff which was welcome; our waiting list was reduced and we were better equipped to cope when staff were on holiday or on sick leave. Later,

I was asked to take a series of weekly classes for nurses, including instruction in lifting techniques and 'keep fit'. They were popular but I was glad to return to working full time with patients.

At this time I started writing papers about my work, having inherited some of Father's journalistic skill; he started his working life as a journalist in London. Having the 'urge' to write really 'fires me' and I need to write down my thoughts directly; it feels as though my brain is working on auto-pilot. My subject matter obviously appealed because several of my articles were published in *Maternal and Child Care* and *My Home and Family*, and later I wrote on the importance of posture from an early age, and breathing exercises.

In the late summer I considered moving to work at Myrtle Street to gain more experience of neonatal physiotherapy. Being near the Women's Hospital it took care of most of the newborn babies that needed paediatric care. The superintendent and staff were very friendly, but unfortunately there was no vacancy for my grade of senior physiotherapist. However Alvon Sausman, a former colleague at Walton and then superintendent physiotherapist at Broadgreen General hospital offered me a job there; I had no hesitation in declining as I so much enjoyed working with children. I later applied for post of deputy superintendent at Alder Hey but due to the lack of applicants, no appointment was made. However when the post was eventually filled we all liked the new deputy and worked well together; she was older than me and had many years' experience in paediatrics.

Social Life

To get to work I drove either along Queen's Drive or more often took the smaller roads across the suburbs of Liverpool. After living at our house in Crosby for a couple of months I regularly passed a neighbour, Tony Lambert, walking up the road. My route passed the gate of Jacob's biscuits factory where I found he worked and thereafter we regularly travelled together. I discovered I knew his fiancée, Angela, and we played squash at the Northern Club. Later, in July 1967, Angela and Tony were married at St Luke's Church in Crosby. Their honeymoon was unusual: they went on a two-year tour around the world, working when they needed to, and stopping in countries they enjoyed. Later I had many holidays with them at their valley home in Branscombe, Devon, and now enjoy hearing news of their family. Mr Rubin, the Superintendent at Alder Hey, also lived in Crosby so we gave each other lifts to and from work when necessary.

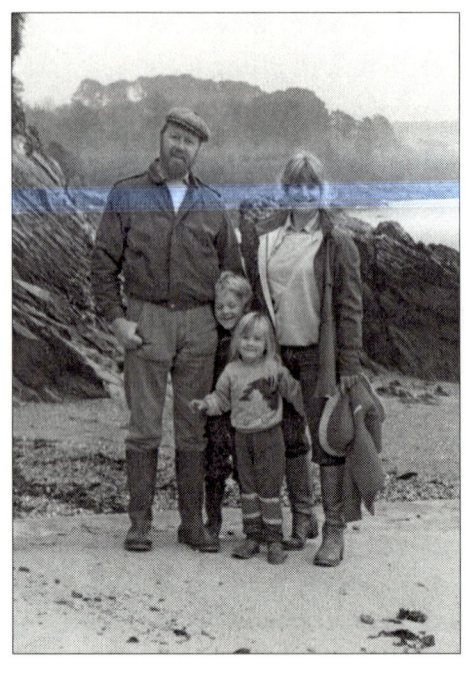

The Lambert family : Angela and Tony with Jamie and Tessa

Some evenings I played tennis on the hospital courts with friends from work or we went out together. Auntie Margaret kept up her contacts in West Derby and I drove her home on many occasions. Twice a week I treated Dorothy Stewart after work trying to ease her pain, and another evening continued helping at West Derby guides. Having my lieutenant's licence I planned to transfer to a company in Crosby as soon as the opportunity arose.

Despite being busy I kept in touch with friends from both schooldays and King's. We were all scattered around the country, but physical distance made no difference to real friendship and I found the old saying 'once a friend, always a friend' was true.

I still found a few people wary when they knew my Father was a bishop but I was proud of him.

Our new house, Cupplesfield, was situated in a quiet residential road about half a mile from the shopping centre of Great Crosby. Most of the houses in the area were of moderate size with generous gardens and the whole area was well wooded; the streets were named after trees, with Cupplesfield in Elm Avenue. We settled quickly, feeling it was a good move, and made friends with neighbours and at our parish church, St Luke's. I joined the Northern Squash club, 100 yards from home, where I played with different members. At weekends I enjoyed bicycling and regularly went to the riverfront at Blundellsands, calling on the Hunton family who I had met at the squash club. I enrolled on the squash club ladder, a knock-out tournament, playing against Angela, my neighbour Tony's fiancée, and also Ann Hardy Smith who played for the county. I always seemed to draw against her in

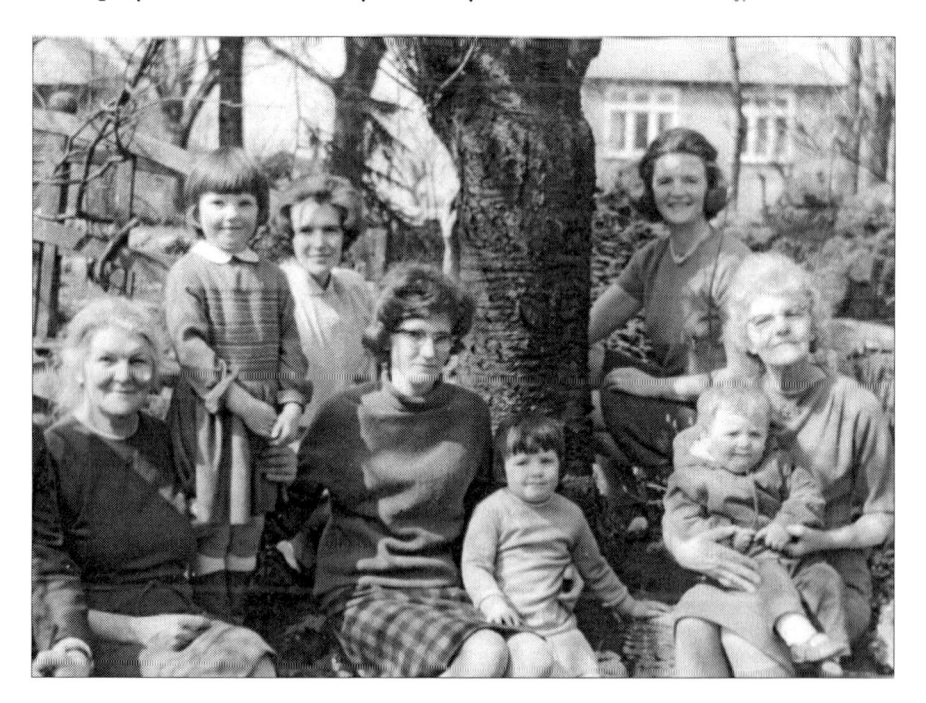

The family in the rockery at Cupplesfield. Left to right My Mother, Sarah, Petrena, Jill, Rachel, Elisabeth and Auntie Margaret with James on her knee

the early rounds of any tournament, but one year I won the 'Plate', a competition for lady members who were eliminated in early rounds of the main tournament.

I also had local boy friends and went to the cinema and dances which were quite fashionable at that time. We met more people when walking Judy, including near neighbours, Sandra Gwyn and her father, who also had a dog. We soon found a good route following a footpath from the end of the road across fields to the wall of Little Crosby estate. The path around the estate passed a field where there were always horses and donkeys, which amused Elisabeth's children when they stayed with us. It was a new experience to live near the countryside as well as the river and we had plenty of choice for walks.

Our house was perfect for visitors; we had plenty of spare bedrooms and large living rooms with an exciting garden and rockery. Elisabeth and her family, who were living near Stockton on Tees, came as often as they could. James, aged two, amused us by pointing to a stone statue of a woman's head on the rockery, and saying 'Mummy', we assumed referring to Elisabeth. The previous owner's son, a landscape designer, had placed stone carvings on the extensive rockery, which had a fountain flowing from rocks into a winding stream. There was only one problem: mares' tail, a most persistent weed, grew abundantly. A wooden bridge provided a good circular route for the children as they chased around the area.

Several colourful, flowering, cherry trees gave shade to the area and in spring I looked down from my bedroom window on to

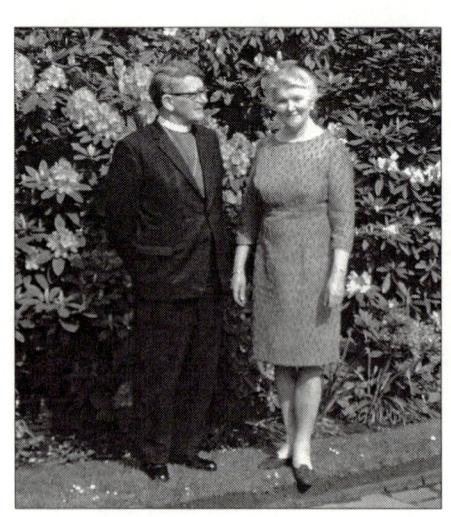

My parents by some of the colourful rhododendrons

the pink blossom. The first year we spent clearing and sorting the large garden. The lawn had been a full sized tennis court and although there was no netting we enjoyed playing, rescuing balls from the rhododendrons. The 'L' shaped house had a paved courtyard with a massive bank of rhododendrons opposite the front door; they were glorious in the early summer and local people came to the entrance to admire the colourful display. There was a double garage opposite the rockery.

Auntie Florrie came often and sometimes brought Daisy, her sister-in-law and husband Fred with her. Cousins visited including Michael who was reading geography at Selwyn College, Cambridge and researching in the Liverpool area, and John Pollock, my boyfriend from London.

Auntie Margaret had a large bedsitting room on the first floor, and a separate kitchen next to ours on the ground floor. She quickly adopted the resident cat Albert; we had agreed to take care of him as the previous owners had moved to a house on a very busy main road. Albert was rather aggressive, so was Judy, our corgi, but an amazing transformation took place when they were in Auntie's sitting room; they would sit side by side on the mat, the only place where they apparently had a 'peace agreement'.

Father didn't have a break when we moved, just a change of address. His secretary, Mrs Margaret Boyd, lived in Formby just north of Crosby; this was convenient as she could call in with papers if he hadn't been to his office in the centre of Liverpool. She became a family friend and after Father's death we corresponded until her death. When coming home from the city Father used the dock road and bought delicious fresh fish from the stalls there.

At Alder Hey we worked alternate Saturday mornings, and were on call for the week-end every five weeks, so had time for some relaxation. Sandra Gwyn encouraged me to attend car maintenance classes again at Crosby school evening institute, but this still proved a bit beyond me. I took up woodwork though, which was an interesting challenge; as my skill improved, table lamps, wooden bowls, bookends and other small pieces were taken home.

The Crosby Guides needed an assistant to help Captain run the company, so a transfer from West Derby was arranged by HQ in Liverpool; the guides were noticeably more noisy than those at West Derby.

Mother and I went to stay for a weekend with Elisabeth and Brian at Billingham; we brought Rachel, aged 3, home with us for a week and she settled happily. Petrena and I enjoyed looking after her and Petrena, having passed her driving test, drove her home.

At Christmas we went to the Cathedral carol services, with the choir and clergy processing up the nave carrying boughs of holly. It was a busy time for Father, and we planned around his commitments. Boxing Day was the day for a long walk, entertaining friends later in the evening.

So 1965 came to an end. I was very happy working at Alder Hey and had achieved my teenage dreams of a career as a hospital paediatric physiotherapist.

The year 1966 started with a very successful party at home for Father's staff to meet socially and see the new diocesan house. It was ideal for entertaining, with a large panelled hall, dining room and lounge, graced with a wide open fireplace, on which sweet chestnuts could be roasted on the burning logs. The kitchen was spacious too with ample surfaces for food preparation; adjoining was a small room with built in wall to ceiling cupboards for china and a hatch through to the dining room.

Early in the summer there was a change in the diocese: Bishop Martin, who had called Father to be his suffragan bishop, retired and the new Bishop, Stuart Blanch, was later enthroned in Liverpool Cathedral. Some years later he became Archbishop of York.

When the evening class syllabus came again, I decided to try my hand at metalwork. We had a good tutor and I enjoyed beating the metal into shape; I made several, good sized, copper plates as presents, as well as ashtrays and small dishes.

During December a group of ordinands came to stay, preparing for ordination to the priesthood. They were reserved and thoughtful at such a time, and had a structured programme of lectures, meditation and prayer, so we had to keep quiet. Living in a bishop's house we accepted this as routine.

Christmas 1966 though was a jolly time spent with family, friends and a Danish physiotherapist from Walton Hospital. After the formal Cathedral service we enjoyed walks, often to Formby a few miles north of Crosby. We trekked through the pine trees and sand dunes looking out for red squirrels, and then on to the vast sandy beach where there always seemed to be strong winds blowing sand into eyes.

Liverpool had a substantial fall of snow in 1968 which was unusual; travel was difficult as the city council weren't used to such weather and their system of road gritting wasn't good, but we managed. A game of squash was an excellent way to get warm.

As winter turned to spring, both Petrena and I decided to change our cars, me to a Fiat 500 which felt safe, and the small engine was very economical with petrol. Friends called it a Noddy car.

In May 1968 another bay of the magnificent Anglican Cathedral in Liverpool was officially opened, and although not regular members of the congregation, we were welcomed. The Cathedral, a vast, lofty building of red brick and stone, always breezy as it was built on one of the few hills in Liverpool, was not completed for another ten years, by which time we lived in Salisbury. Petrena was able to come too. She had a good position in charge of the children's department at Crosby Library where she arranged a number of successful activities.

Holidays

During the summer Margaret and John Statham, friends of Auntie Margaret, who had worked with her at Abbots'

Bromley School in Staffordshire, invited me to stay on their farm near Uttoxeter. They had three young children and days were spent helping with the animals or exploring the farm. John invited me to drive sheep to Uttoxeter market, and Margaret took me to some of the countryside surrounding the small market town, serving local farms of varying acreage, set in an attractive area with mile upon mile of gently undulating hills.

Holiday at Swan Lake cottage

AFTER REPEATED INVITATIONS from Tony and Madeline Stroud, whom Father had met the previous year when leading a pilgrimage to the Holy Land, to stay at their cottage at Higher Coombe, near Shaftesbury in Dorset, we decided to accept, and returned regularly for the next thirty years. The cottage was small and situated on the banks of a 3-acre lake which the family also owned and on which visitors could use their boats. We went via Cambridge where Father had work to attend to and I stayed with a school friend, Prue Murphy (née Green) again. After the bleakness of Salisbury Plain, the scenery changed to rolling hills and wooded valleys. When we turned off the main road towards Higher Coombe the narrow lane dipped down to a valley covered in treetops, with no sign of a lake or habitation. Cautiously we drove on among huge beech and coniferous trees and after a hairpin bend came to another steep hill lined with banks of tall trees behind rhododendrons. After a collection of cottages and a lake the lane narrowed and suddenly we saw another lake and an attractive cottage with a swan symbol in the low thatched roof.

The pink colourwashed cottage with four rooms was an old, single storey stone building, with an exterior chimney stack, and a more recently added extension at the rear. The two thatched porch doors, and windows between, looked out to the lake. The cottage and garden were on a lower level than the road, with treacherous

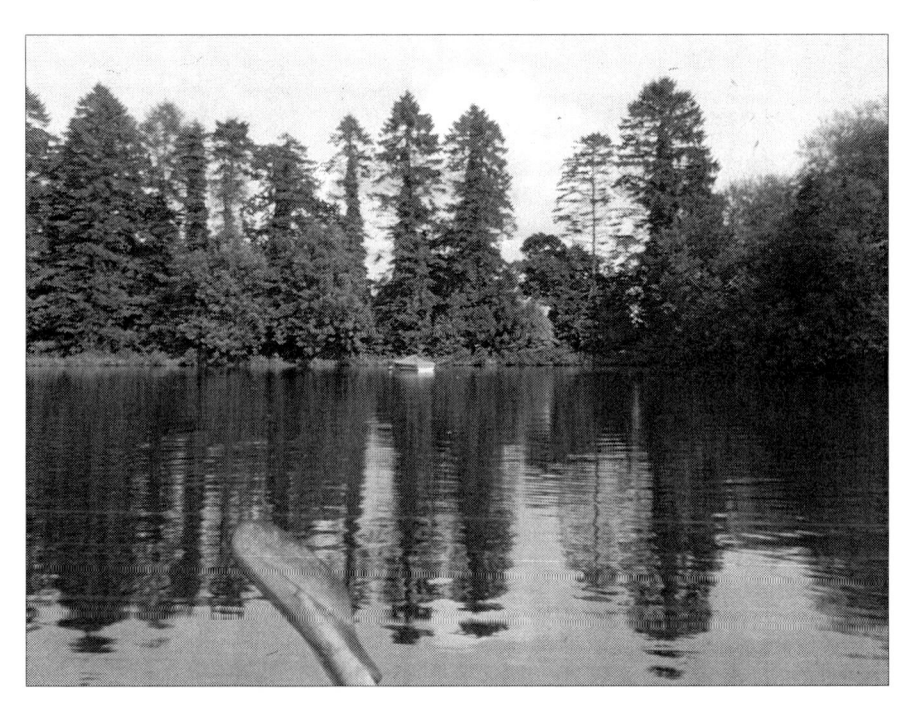

Swan Lake

steps down to the small colourful garden, and a small apple orchard beyond. A huge sycamore tree overshadowed the lawn, and several brightly painted boats were pulled up in front of the cottage. The lake, with clumps of water lilies scattered on the surface, extended into the distance, with trees and bamboo on its banks. The only sounds were the small waterfall filling the lake, bird song, and wind in the trees.

A path ran round the near side of the lake to the deep end; the family punt was moored at a landing stage a short distance from the house. An out-fall led to another lake in the next field; the far bank was tightly wooded, with bamboos and reeds. The lake was fed by a noisy inlet of water which came under the road from a spring that was the source of the river Nadder, eventually flowing into the Avon at Salisbury, where we moved in 1977 and where the Strouds had their main house.

The cottage had originally been three very small, adjoining farm cottages, which were converted at the turn of the 20th century

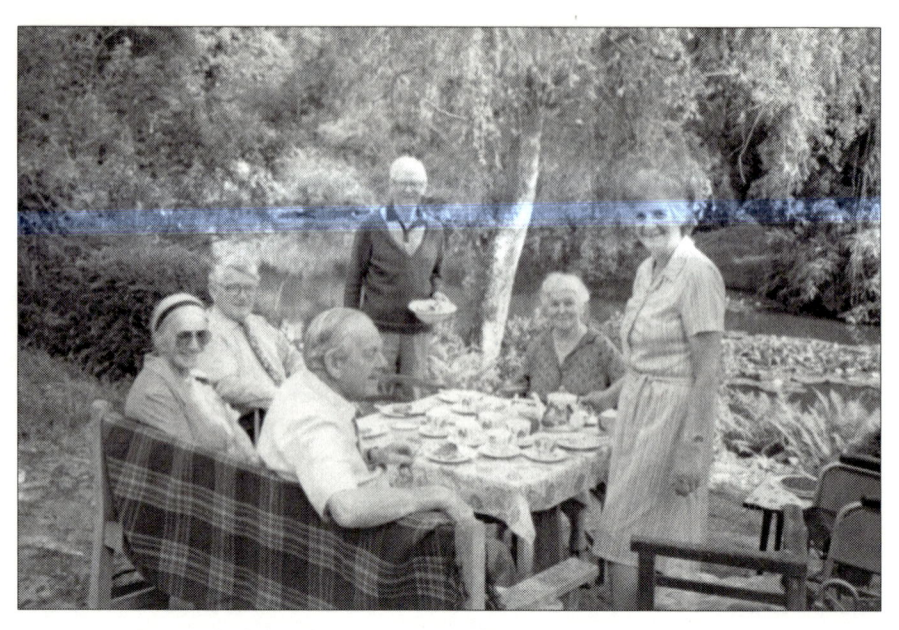

Tea on the lakeside with Tony and Madeline Stroud and guests

when bathroom and toilet were added at the back. The interior was comfortable; high ceilings in the living and dining rooms lent an air of spaciousness and the smell of years of wood fires from the open grate gave a friendly, homely aroma. The living room doubled as a second bedroom and at bedtime the flickering light of the embers in the fireplace was comforting. The dining/kitchen room was decorated with Swiss plates hanging on the walls.

Here there was a second doorway to the garden which made easy access to a picnic table, from which kingfishers could be seen on the lake. The main bedroom was up four wooden stairs and led to the bathroom which backed on to the orchard. Outside a garden shed contained gardening equipment, oars and seats for the boats; there was also a log shed and a summer house, with more seats and cushions for the punt.

Madeline, the main gardener of the family, had planted shrubs and bushes which, with the tall long established deciduous and coniferous trees, surrounded the lake and kept it well protected from winds. The orchard provided apples for autumn visits, whereas during the summer we collected wild strawberries and blackberries from the hedgerows. The peaceful atmosphere was in striking contrast to our life in industrial Liverpool, and we knew we would be happy here.

During our first visit the weather was fine, dry and warm and Father and I swam in the lake daily. Madeline believed the water had healing properties and it was certainly refreshing and invigorating. We tried fishing for trout from boats, which we were advised was more successful than lakeside fishing. Mother, being nervous of water, at first felt unsafe in a small boat, but soon forgot her fears and became an expert fisherwoman, and Father learnt the art of preparing the fish for cooking in the cottage oven.

Shaftesbury was our nearest local town, a fascinating place with narrow streets and panoramic views over the surrounding countryside from the famous Gold Hill. It had been built as a hill town, with a steep drop from the remains of an Abbey on the western summit. Fish and chips from the shop in the high street were the best we had tasted, and a bakery made Dorset lardy cake, a favourite of Father's.

We had plenty of incentive to go walking, for apart from collecting fruit there were many paths and lanes to explore in the wooded valley, with the Rising Sun pub about half a mile away. Beyond the cottage there were another five or so houses on the hillside, and above the hamlet a Roman Catholic Girls' boarding school. The path to the school was lined with rhododendrons. We met some of our neighbours, and Uncle Roland and Aunt Ruth from Dorchester, with any of their family who were at home, also visited. I had my first sight of a kingfisher there, and every time I see one I gasp at the beauty and strong colours of these small birds with their speedy flight. Deer visited the lakeside; we had to keep a watch for young deer who liked to eat the saplings which the Strouds had planted. Badgers were also present in the area.

My parents and I returned to Swan Lake Cottage for another holiday later that year and introduced Petrena, who joined us, to the cottage, boating and walks. It was August and we had good weather, so my Father and I bathed and we all went out in the boats: I preferred the canoe while my parents and Petrena fished from the punt. They caught rainbow trout, and on the last day Petrena, who was a successful fisherwoman, persuaded me to help so she could catch a fish to take home for Auntie Margaret. Although I disliked killing fish by hitting them on the head with the tool called 'the priest', and was squeamish about gutting and eating them, I managed.

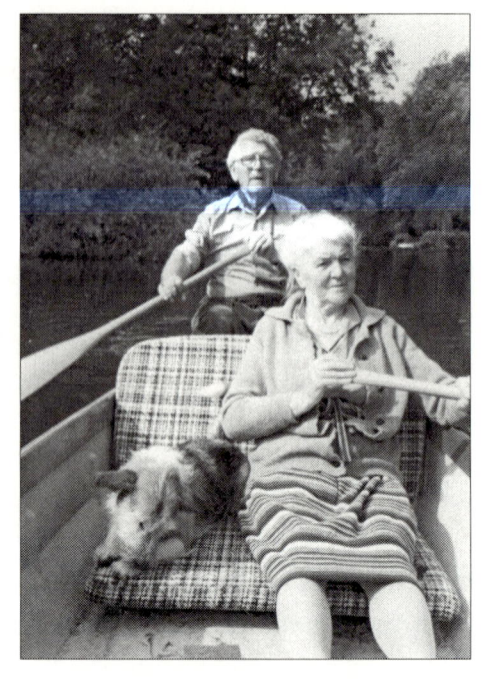

My parents with Suki in the punt at Swan Lake

The local vicar was an old friend of Father's and invited him to officiate at his church. We went to Salisbury to shop and to visit the Strouds there. The weather was usually good, but an open log fire in the sitting room, reading or playing board games, compensated for any rain.

Later in the year I had another holiday when the Stathams invited me to stay on the farm again and Auntie Margaret joined me for the end of the week.

In 1968 I had an early summer holiday with Elisabeth and her family at a cottage belonging to the Diocese in Hawkshead in the Lake District. We had a wonderful time exploring the area, walking and climbing. The views from the summit of the mountains were splendid and I felt on top of the world. Sarah and Rachel were good walkers but James still needed encouragement and sometimes a ride on his father's shoulders. We revisited friends in Grasmere, and made friends with

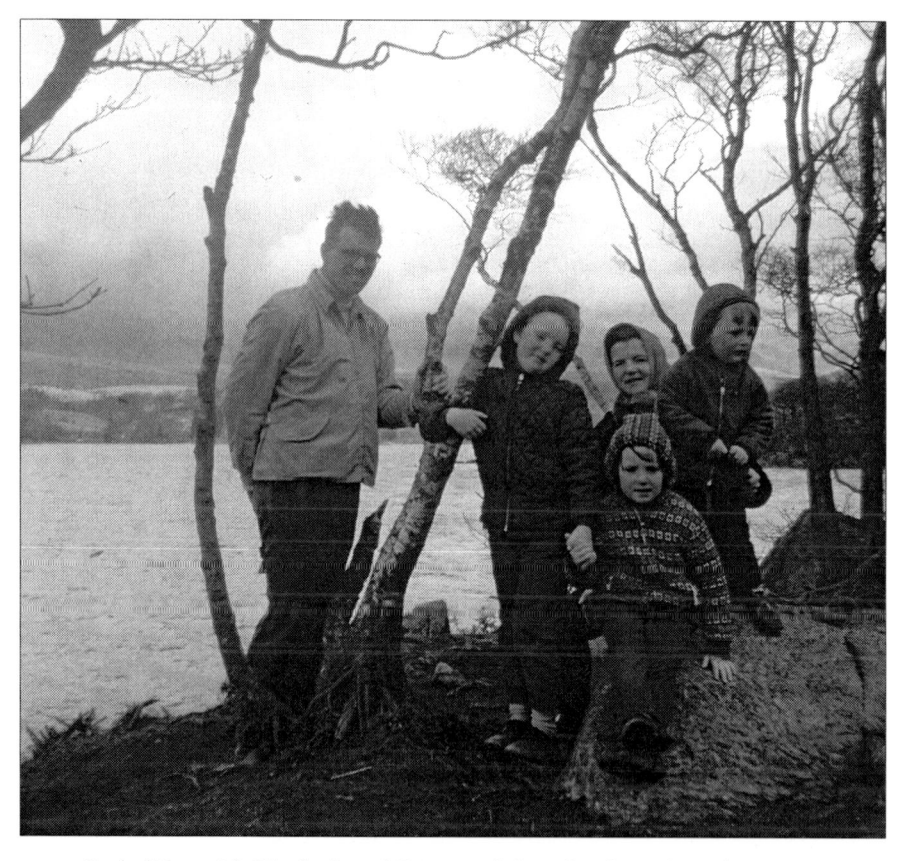

On holiday with Elisabeth and Brian and their family in the Lake District

the local farmer and his young family. The girls enjoyed horse riding with Elisabeth, but I preferred walking in the fells or by the Lakes: I always enjoyed being near water.

Personal Health

IN THE WINTER and early months of 1966 the team was very busy treating babies and children with the usual winter chest problems. I myself had repeated sinus infections, common in Liverpool with the damp, salty atmosphere, and working in the midst of a multitude of germs didn't help. Back pains recurred but didn't keep me from work.

During the spring of 1966 I developed a deep, antibiotic-resistant infection in one of my fingernails and it wasn't safe to work with sick children. Eventually the infection proved so resistant that I had an operation on the nail bed which cured the problem. My GP, Dr Webster, also treated recurrent digestive problems but apart from a couple of days off work after the operation I kept working, though was noticeably more tired for social activities.

Late in the year I was off work several times with throat and chest infections again leading to sinusitis. Increasing backache and recurrent stomach pains also troubled me. Apart from having time off work, I couldn't enjoy my social life; squash matches and outings with friends had to be postponed. I went to see Dr G E Honey, a gastroenterologist at Broadgreen Hospital; I had previously seen him privately. He eventually diagnosed spasm in my stomach and bowel, to be managed with medication and small regular meals, sometimes awkward when working but snacks overcame the problem if meals were delayed.

By the summer of 1967 my health had deteriorated and Dr Honey altered the medication for my gastro-intestinal spasm, hoping this would improve my digestion and persistent fatigue, despite regular meals and supplements of milk drinks and yoghurt. In addition, a fast-moving squash ball severely bruised one of my knees, and soon after I received another hard blow to my right wrist, causing severe pain. Mr Dwyer, orthopaedic surgeon, suggested strapping my wrist and thought it would recover within a few months. I carried on working, although the painful wrist made it difficult as our work was all 'hands on' and physical.

During the autumn sinusitis troubled me again, complicated by severe nosebleeds. I was referred back to Mr Pracy, the ENT surgeon, with an acute sinus infection and had regular appointments during the following years with repeated cauterisation, and different drugs were prescribed. My joints also rebelled against the damp weather, but I carried on working, hoping all would improve with drier weather.

By June 1968 my right wrist, injured the previous year playing squash, had become more painful. Although I had by then trained myself to write and play squash left handed to ease the load on my right wrist, working was painful and difficult. Eventually I had to return to the orthopaedic department at Alder Hey. Mr Walkden, a Registrar, injected the wrist with hydrocortisone and later partly immobilised it with strapping. This produced little benefit so a plaster of paris cast was applied for two weeks which effectively relieved the pain. However when this was removed the wrist was again very painful. A special X-Ray showed that the small disc lying between the two forearm bones was torn, an unusual injury. Mr Walkden suggested an operation might be necessary if the pain didn't improve in another four weeks.

There was no improvement and my left wrist also began to ache. A firm wrist support was to be used long term, and further strain was to be avoided, so no more metalwork or woodwork, nor strenuous games of squash. I was worried that the best of my working days as a physiotherapist might be over.

8
The Rot Sets In ~ 1968-69

Introduction

THE WRIST SUPPORT on my right arm meant adapting my working methods but I managed to treat all my patients, though arriving home tired and ready for relaxation. Colleagues at metalwork were very supportive, and, determined that my work would be completed, hammered and moulded metal for me. By the end of the year I had made wrought iron candleholders, a fireguard and umbrella stand, and several beaten copper plates and ashtrays. Squash defeated me even using skill rather than strength – the pain in my wrists took away the pleasure of playing.

Knitting aggravated my wrists so I concentrated on dressmaking, with help from Auntie Margaret; according to her and Mother my sewing looked clumsy but the results were successful.

Personal Health

BY THE SPRING both my wrists were causing more pain and my elbows and neck had also become painful, so I returned to the orthopaedic registrar. He thought the cartilage between the two forearm bones in my right wrist was torn, and recommended that I see Mr Osbourne, a consultant orthopaedic surgeon at the Royal Liverpool Hospital. I also went back to Dr Honey at Broadgreen as my digestive problems had increased, and further bouts of sinusitis resulted in yet more severe nosebleeds requiring repeated cauterisation and antibiotics from Mr Pracey, the ENT Consultant.

Mr Osbourne diagnosed carpal tunnel syndrome and injected my right hand, but unfortunately this didn't relieve the pain. Tests on my stomach again showed a problem with the lining of the digestive system and spasm in the stomach and bowels, for which more medication was prescribed.

In March 1969 Mr Osbourne, told me I might have early rheumatoid arthritis or early signs of Keinboch's disease, a serious degenerative bone disease (osteochondritis) of one of the small bones in the hand. A leather cock up splint was provided to keep the right wrist supported in a good position. I found it possible to continue working by using my left arm, but that gave extra strain on my already weakened left wrist. Squash had become impossible.

Early in May, after months of pain and difficulty doing my work, Dr Webster, my GP, referred me to Mr Beddow, an orthopaedic surgeon at Whiston Hospital, near Liverpool, for a second opinion. Within a few days an exploratory operation of the right wrist confirmed a pathological tear of the suspect cartilage; this was removed and the wrist never seized up again. By experience, my immediate reaction when it 'locked' was to give traction, which would unlock it; that was now a thing of the past. The operating staff found it difficult to wake me after the anaesthetic; the first of several times I had similar problems. Later X rays of my left wrist showed a suspected chip off one of the bones but Mr Beddow suggested leaving this until the right wrist was back to full use. Fortunately dexterity using my left hand had improved for dressing, eating and writing, so I was able to put pen to paper again, typing my latest piece about my work with children with cerebral palsy. 'Cerebral Palsy: A Physiotherapist's approach' was published in *Maternal and Child Care* in October 1971. I went back to work after three weeks but found it tiring and difficult, as my right wrist was still weak; wax baths and exercises were added to the treatment.

Early in July American astronauts landed on the moon, a major breakthrough in space travel. Soon after, my parents and I started to prepare for a week's holiday in Majorca – my first time of flying and a holiday abroad; a passport and injections were needed. Within days of our final injections my parents were sick. They recovered quickly, then I had vomiting and severe stomach pains; appendicitis or a virus infection was suspected. It turned out that we had food poisoning which was traced to a joint of ham purchased from a local butcher. The accompanying diarrhoea exacerbated my colonic irritability, which was a life long problem. We soon improved and were able to leave for Luton airport and stayed overnight with Auntie Florrie who lived nearby.

After the holiday my stomach problems persisted and Dr Honey diagnosed a recurrence of colitis, which required drug treatment. By now, with regular visits to the GP and hospitals, I was beginning to experience what it was to be 'on the other side', and didn't like it.

Mr Beddow suggested ultrasound for adhesions in the right wrist and both elbows, which he thought had developed 'golfer's elbow'. This didn't relieve the pain, so the day before we moved to Birmingham in late December, I returned for the first of many hydrocortisone injections. I was worried that I would not be able to continue my work.

Work

AT THE HOSPITAL we had a large and cheerful porter, Jimmy, to transport patients from the wards to our department. He was tactful and polite, and his sense of humour with the children eased their worries; he was always willing and had a heart of gold.

We were always busy but when I was off sick other members of staff looked after patients on my wards, though no one treated my patients at the Spastic Centre; so parents had to continue their child's exercises to prevent development of contractures and strengthen muscles.

The summer of 1968 alternated between cold wet periods and intensely hot days when the Spastic Centre became intolerably hot and we took the children on to the small patch of grass just outside. I was extremely busy during my limited sessions and really needed an assistant so Mr Rubin asked management for extra staff.

As Christmas approached the Spastic Centre held its annual party. The children were so excited and it was good to see them with their families; brothers and sisters usually caused more problems than they did. Jean, our orderly, helped us transform the treatment rooms into a colourful playroom, and the catering department provided delicious refreshments.

When I was off work, Dorothy Stewart missed her treatment. When I returned, her older sister, Catherine, was a patient at Park House Nursing Home in Crosby so I treated her as well as Dorothy who was at home. Their rheumatoid arthritis was very unstable and their health varied from day to day, but I did all I could to help them, and passed messages between the two. Over Christmas 1968 I was asked to treat patients privately at Park House for the first time. I couldn't fully commit myself, having enough to do at Alder Hey and with my two private patients, but agreed to treat occasional patients with acute chest conditions.

My young private patient, M, (who had cerebral palsy) went away for a holiday with his family, which noticeably benefited his general health, enabling me to start new exercises for the next stages of his physical development. He began to roll himself over, and although this was months after his twin sister, it was the start of his independent movement. He was obviously delighted with the freedom and chuckled with pleasure, even though he couldn't speak. On returning to work after my operation I found he was sitting unsupported for 30 seconds. We worked to improve his balance and further strengthen his muscles, and I had a small chair and table designed and made-to-measure to enable him to sit, and therefore encourage him to use his hands purposefully. In the New Year I asked a colleague who also worked with children with cerebral palsy to make a joint visit to M, as it was always good to have a second opinion. Later that year my next paper, on 'The value of Physiotherapy for children', was published in *Maternal and Child Care*.

When we eventually moved to Birmingham in December 1969 I was sorry to be leaving Alder Hey and my private patients after seven years. Several former patients corresponded after we left and it was a joy to hear that the boy with Guillain Barré syndrome was running around and behaving like a normal child.

Holiday

My parents and I set off to Swan Lake Cottage again in summer 1968 going via Gloucester, where we spent the weekend with Reggie Houghton, Father's former secretary at Southwark, and visited other Southwark friends who had retired to the area. Reggie had joined the staff of Gloucester Cathedral and lived in the Close, also having responsibility for some small, medieval city churches. I explored the town centre, particularly the fine Cathedral with examples of architecture dating from Norman to early Perpendicular, and attended Sunday services. After three days we left for Wiltshire. Apart from essential shopping in Shaftesbury, exploring Win Green, part of the old sheep drove across the downs from Shaftesbury to Salisbury, and an evening with the Stroud's at their home in Salisbury, we spent all our time at the cottage. I visited the Cathedral and Close for the first time, not knowing we would move within walking distance of the Cathedral in years to come.

When bathing at Swan Lake Cottage we either had to walk along the lakeside, or take the punt to the far end where the water was about twenty-foot deep. Stone steps from the retaining wall went down into the water and beyond the steps the bank was interrupted by a narrow waterfall whence the lake water poured down to the lower level of the next stream. This stream subsequently flowed into the third of the chain of lakes along the Nadder valley before going on to Salisbury. A row of stately trees marked the boundary of Swan Lake cottage grounds just beyond the end of the lake, and it was an attractive setting for a bathe – open to the skies and with coots and moorhens making their croaking noise. The fish favoured the deep end of the lake where there was a lot of weed; I dreaded getting tangled in it or touching a fish but that apart loved our swims there. We chose the time by the sun as that obviously affected the water temperature, which was usually refreshing rather than warm, but floating in such idyllic surroundings under a clear blue sky was a delight. I hoped that the water would help my aches and pains, but in fact canoeing and punting were too strenuous for comfort. If it was at all chilly in the evenings we lit the wood fire using logs cut from trees around the lake: the aroma gave the whole cottage a special fragrance.

I mentioned that we went to Majorca in July 1969. We stayed at Villa Mimosa with Mother's school friend from Luton days, Ethel Morris and her husband Frank. The flight was exciting and good, apart from intense pain in my ears on take off and landing at Palma. We collected a hire car to drive north east to Pollensa and the villa, named after the colourful shrubs outside the property. The holiday was a great success: Father and I usually bathed in the warm sea twice a day at local beaches, and we shopped

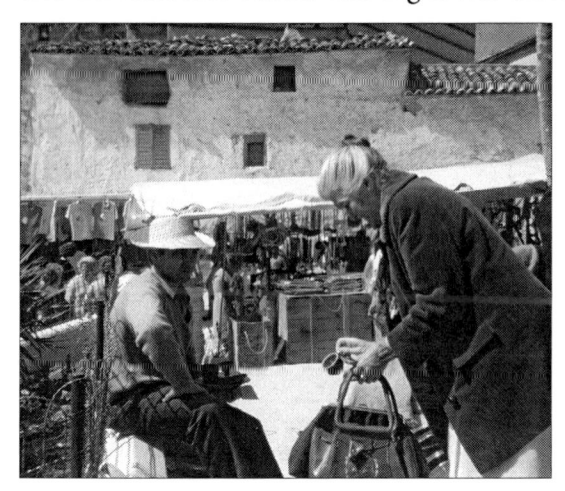

Mother bargaining with a stall holder in Pollensa market, Majorca

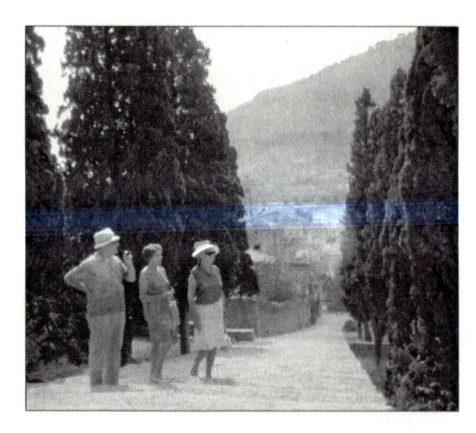

Pollensa- a steep path up from the village– Father with my Mother and Auntie Ethel

in the fascinating old town with its narrow, cobbled streets, Mother buying numerous souvenirs. We climbed to the local hilltop monastery where we had marvellous panoramic views of the countryside, and walked among the fields past little 'thinkas' (smallholdings) where owners grew vegetables, produced for their own consumption and for taking to market; we collected fruits, including blackberries and figs, growing wild in the hedgerows. The windmills fascinated me, as well as the sight of farmers leading bullocks to pull ploughs and till the soil; it felt as though the clocks had been turned back a century. Father and I attended Mass in Pollensa and watched young children dressed like brides filing into the splendid Italianate building.

While at the villa we experienced a most violent thunderstorm. Pollensa is surrounded by mountainous hills on three sides and the flashes of lightning streaked across the sky from one side of the valley to the other, then seemed to bounce back again, as did the terrific claps of thunder. Fascinated by storms, Father watched from the verandah, while I crouched inside. It certainly cleared the air, for the next days were bright and sunny. Sometimes we had meals at Porta Pollensa about a mile from the old town, where we watched local food being cooked on spits in the cafés.

We drove to the mountains in the north east of the island where the roads were frightening, with hairpin bends on steep hills with a sheer drop to the side, and reckless drivers going extremely fast. In our small hire car we drove cautiously: the scenery was fabulous and the tremendous views across the mountains and down to the coast with the deep blue sea beyond remain a memory.

✻ *The Rot Sets In* ✻

Social Life

During the autumn of 1968 I met Gordon, who played squash and cricket at the Northern Squash Club. We started to go out several times a week to the cinema, dances or meals, as well as socialising at the squash club. His parents invited me to their home for meals and he came to Cupplesfield and met my parents. We went to opera, the excellent Royal Liverpool Philharmonic orchestra, and to plays at the Royal Court theatre as well as enjoying several dinner dances. He was very tolerant and taught me more about dancing than the classes that we'd had as children. I was often not in bed till after midnight which was most unusual for me.

We had snow again that Christmas, but fortunately it didn't linger. Our home was full as Elisabeth and her family with her parents-in-law stayed, but with plenty of adults to share the cooking and inevitable washing up, we all enjoyed ourselves. Cupplesfield was large enough to be able to entertain the extended family, and Gordon came to a meal to meet all my family, which went well. It was the custom at Liverpool to hold a carol service after Christmas, which was unusual at that time, and we all thoroughly enjoyed the choir's singing. However soon after the New Year, Gordon and I parted; he was serious about our relationship and wanted commitment, but I was too keen on my work and career.

After enjoying a week's holiday at home before the early Easter when Elisabeth and family stayed with us, we had a major surprise: Father was invited to become Bishop in South Australia. This was tempting and at first we were all excited at the prospect. I spoke to some Australians who worked at Alder Hey and they were enthusiastic about life there, but after the initial excitement, reality supervened, with hesitation about moving to such a distant country. Father, as usual when he had a major decision to make, lost his appetite. I had to make up my own mind about such a big move and the effect on my career and life in general. Petrena was quick to decide not to leave England, and by the time Father announced that he would not accept the invitation, I had determined not to move, so life returned to normal.

During the summer I saw more of my local friends socially, and regularly cycled to see Shirley Hunton, from the squash club, and her boys in Blundellsands. From their home I went on to the shore, a favourite place to watch the large ships go up and down the Mersey estuary, for Liverpool was a busy port at that time. There was always a refreshing breeze there. Gordon came back into my life and would come round to our home, but we were just good friends. My dressmaking flourished: I was able to make dresses, blouses and skirts, choosing material and patterns at Ormskirk market, where there were several stalls selling good quality materials at reasonable prices.

Move to Birmingham

THREE DAYS AFTER our return from Majorca Father told us he had been invited to be the Bishop of Birmingham and felt he should accept. Petrena and I now had to decide if we wanted to remain in Liverpool and find our own homes or move to Birmingham and get new jobs. The house, called Bishop's Croft, was large with seven bedrooms and a separate flat on the third floor, and there was a vast garden; Father would have a secretary, and a chauffeur and gardener with houses in the grounds. Auntie Margaret regretted leaving Liverpool and her friends, especially Freda Critchley, but quickly decided she would like the flat in return for help with the house and garden. Petrena was happy in her job as children's librarian at the new library in Crosby and decided to stay until she found a comparable post in Birmingham; Freda immediately offered her a home for as long as she wanted. I decided to find a job in Birmingham and move with my parents.

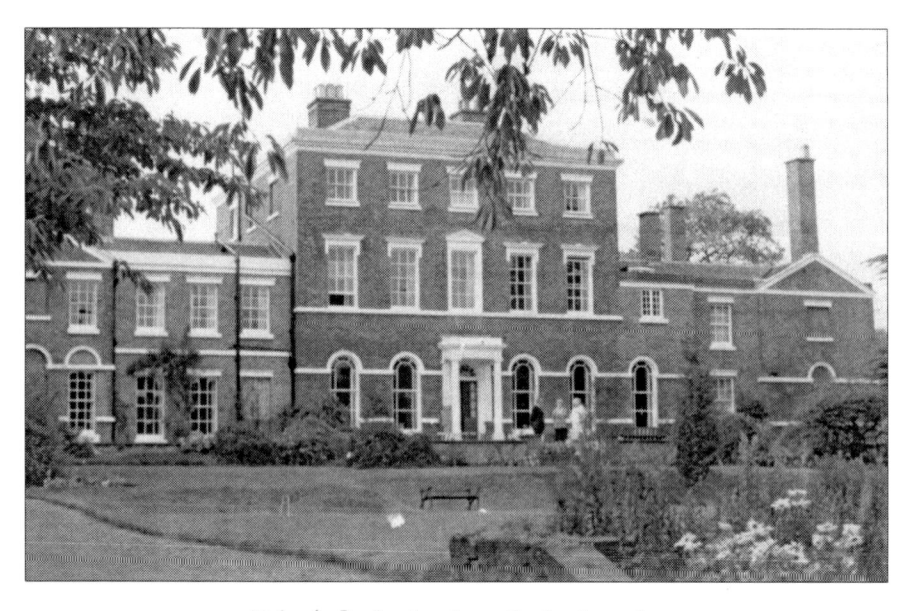

Bishop's Croft, view from the back garden

My application for a job at Birmingham Childrens' Hospital, about four miles from our new home, was successful after an interview at the small, rather old-fashioned hospital in Edgbaston. Bishop's Croft was in the pleasant suburb of Harborne on the south west side of Birmingham. It had a central, three-storey block with a two-storey building either side, set back in extensive grounds near the main outer ring road of Birmingham, and approached from a side road which bordered a field belonging to the property which provided grazing for horses. Harborne Cricket Club occupied another side, and a path to Church House, where Father's secretary and official office would be, on the remaining side. A chapel had been added which Father used daily, and shared with colleagues who came for meetings or to stay. The Church Commissioners, who owned the house, had decided to convert one wing into a self contained flat to be rented out by them on a commercial basis.

Soon after the appointment was announced we were hounded by press and television reporters as Father had been a popular figure in Liverpool. He was to succeed Bishop Leonard Wilson, well known nationally for his appearances at the Remembrance Day services at the Royal Albert Hall, having been a prisoner of war in Singapore during the Second World War. The position was important, for Birmingham was proud of being Britain's second city, and although small in size, the diocese had a very large population, mainly in the city area. Even in the late 1960s there was a considerable ethnic mix which posed a significant challenge. Father was to take up his duties at the beginning of 1970.

My good-byes to staff and patients including Dorothy Stewart and M were made before Christmas. My final duty should have been the last Saturday of December 1969, but on the Sunday morning I was needed to treat an acutely ill child and again returned later that evening. I wasn't going to be allowed to leave till the very end. The same day Mother was injured: on Father's final Sunday duty at a parish church, she fell over, and we thought had sprained her ankle. The ankle became extremely swollen, and I applied the usual first aid. She assured me it would be all right, so we left Liverpool on a very cold December 31st. I drove down the motorway in my Fiat 500 with Judy the dog for company, all set for the next stage of life in Birmingham.

9
To Birmingham

We arrived at Bishop's Croft on the evening of December 31st 1969 to find chaos. The builders were working and throughout the ground floor rooms half the floorboards were missing; Mother's ankle had swollen greatly during the journey and she couldn't put weight on her leg because of pain; and the press arrived to take our photographs. The removal men took two days to unpack which wasn't surprising as they had to avoid the workmen and climb around floorboards, as well as find their way around the large house. We kept them happy with constant supplies of tea and cakes and they were remarkably good humoured about the whole situation.

What a start to life in Birmingham.

Elisabeth and Brian, who moved from Stockton on Tees to St Albans in Hertfordshire at this time, were in the same predicament and we couldn't help with their three young children.

We quickly called the local GP, Dr Alan Pearce, recommended by the previous bishop; suspecting a broken ankle he sent Mother for an X ray. Fortunately Father's chauffeur was available so he took her while Father started work at his nearby office, leaving Petrena, Auntie Margaret and myself to get the house in better order. Mother returned on crutches with her leg in a below knee plaster and not allowed to put any weight on it, tricky when negotiating missing floorboards. Exploring the cellar, I fell awkwardly, bruising my arms and legs, which wasn't helpful; we didn't use the cellar after that.

The Church Commissioners were responsible for furnishing the main rooms used for official functions, and these were almost ready for use. We concentrated on the bedrooms and finding homes for our own furniture. My bedsitting room was light and very large with views over the chapel, the small courtyard and back garden, while Petrena chose a smaller room in the centre of the house next to my parents' bedroom, where there was a plaque stating the Prince of Wales had slept there in the 1930s.

There was a heavy fall of snow during those first few days and as Bishop's Croft is on high ground and very exposed, we found it extremely cold. Father's chauffeur, Alfred Turland, was most helpful in directing Petrena and me to the shops and Birmingham Childrens' Hospital, when I started work the following week, and we explored the local shops in Harborne and stocked up food cupboards, realising Mother wouldn't be able to get out for a few weeks. Petrena had a successful interview at West Bromwich library to start work in March.

We prepared the house for relatives who were to stay the following weekend to attend Father's magnificent enthronement as fifth Bishop of Birmingham. Mother was indignant at having to go in a wheelchair. The Cathedral staff had organised lunch for all the family, including our cousins who had travelled from around the country to be present; afterwards most of them returned to view our new home, and Elisabeth and family stayed the weekend.

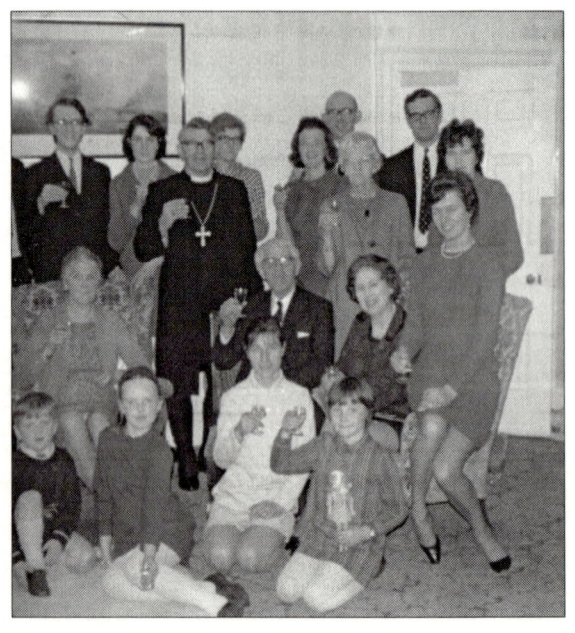

The family celebration at Bishop's Croft after Father's enthronement as Bishop of Birmingham at the Cathedral

✳ *To Birmingham* ✳

Bishop's Croft

ONE WING OF the house accommodated Father's large study, which led, via a small walled garden, to his private chapel which he used for daily prayers. The chapel was also available for the regular staff meetings and for other services when Father had visiting clergy or ordinands. Auntie Margaret offered to be responsible for the cleaning which relieved Mother of one responsibility.

The north facing front of the house, which had originally been the back, as was obvious from all the drainpipes on that side, had a large walled, formal garden opposite with colourful rose bushes set among grassed areas, and a vegetable garden including a spacious greenhouse on the right. Originally open fields surrounded the house but Harborne Cricket Club had purchased the field to the north of the front garden some years before from the Church Commissioners. Church House where the diocesan staff had offices was built on the east, and the field to the west, rented out by the Church Commissioners, provided grazing for horses.

John our gardener had a Glaswegian wife and two young children who would greet us when we parked our cars in the garage adjacent to their house and north west of Bishop's Croft.

The garden door at the back of our house opened on to a paved terrace overlooking an extensive lawn, with gracious coniferous trees providing shade on the east. We enjoyed meals on the terrace, weather permitting. The lawn was large enough for a tennis court but in the absence of netting we played croquet and clock golf instead. During the summer we entertained parties from the Diocese and abroad, as well as having annual tea parties for clergy and their wives.

The house had been built and owned by a wealthy city businessman, who made his money from the metal trade, and had high, elegant moulded ceilings which suited it perfectly. The front door opened into a large room-sized hall which was just high enough to accommodate the grandfather clock with a friendly chime given to Father by his friend, Eric Evans, the Archdeacon of Southport on the latter's retirement. I have it to this day. The dining room was oak panelled throughout, lightened by long windows overlooking the paved terrace area and garden. It had a steel fireplace, useful to supplement central heating in winter, and with a long oval dining table and matching chairs the room looked elegant. The official lounge, also with moulded ceilings and long windows on to the back garden, had a fine decorated Adam fireplace set in a tiled hearth. This room could be extended using a shuttered partition to include a small family sitting room.

Work

THE MONDAY AFTER Father's enthronement I started work and met the staff of the Children's Hospital: the Superintendent, Miss V. Naylor, and three basic grade staff who showed me round. Our department was a small prefabricated building on the edge of the site (a new hospital has since been built.) The hospital included orthopaedic, general medical and surgical departments and also the Midlands Centre for children's cardio-thoracic (heart and lung) disease. I hadn't treated such patients before, but after working with colleagues, I soon had my own patients and watched operations. It amazed me that the babies and young children tolerated such procedures and then bounced back to health in a relatively short time. Some babies needed operations on their first day of life; they were so tiny and delicate that we used finger pressure only to vibrate their chests and clear the lungs of any infections and secretions. Others were seriously ill, with some on life support machines for prolonged periods, having been born with a heart or lung defect.

The commonest congenital heart lesion was patent ductus

arteriosus where the junction between the aorta and pulmonary artery fails to close, thus putting an extra load on the left ventricle. Next were atrial or ventricular septal defects allowing blood to shunt between the chambers, and then pulmonary stenosis when the valve becomes thickened and reduces blood flow through the lungs. The latter could be an isolated defect or, more seriously, associated with other congenital lesions, known as Tetralogy of Fallot.

The hospital was also the regional centre for cystic fibrosis, an inherited disease where secretions from the lining of the lungs are thick and tenacious causing repeated chest infections. They require daily lifelong chest physiotherapy of postural drainage and percussion to aid removal of the secretions from the lungs, and when suffering an infection this must be done several times each day. We treated them on the wards and taught the parents how to perform treatment at home. Sometimes the children attended as outpatients if they were having problems, and when older they learnt to drain themselves and do exercises to loosen sputum. Often they also lacked a digestive enzyme usually manufactured by the pancreas, causing malabsorption, unless treated with the replacement enzyme.

I soon had my own list of general ward patients, some recovering from operations, as well as regular outpatients, many with orthopaedic conditions, cerebral palsy and spina bifida, and took turns for being on call for intensive care. We seemed to have a wider range of background and nationalities than in Liverpool; Indian and Asian patients were often accompanied by an English speaking relation, often a child, who acted as translator, because the parents did not speak English. I got used to treating tiny babies whose bodies smelt of curry, spices and garlic, which was carried not only in their breath and clothes but in the pores of their skin. As at Alder Hey the balance of treating children who made good recoveries from their illness charged my enthusiasm for treating those with chronic diseases such as cerebral palsy (a term that has replaced 'spastic' which only describes one type).

In August, 1970, after working for eight months, I was promoted to a new senior grade post, the same as at Alder Hey. In 1971 an article of mine called 'Cerebral Palsy: a Physiotherapist's approach' was published in *Maternal and Child Care* and a few weeks later reported by the *Birmingham Post*, together with a photograph of my work with a patient. The consultant who looked after children with cerebral palsy was also involved in the interview and the report stimulated much interest. Later that year we had students in their final year of training from the Queen Elizabeth Hospital School of Physiotherapy; I found this teaching stimulating and in 1973 when my health deteriorated, it proved a good way of using my knowledge without the physical exertion of treating patients.

Social Life

I MET UP SOCIALLY with Sue Philp (neé Bastable) and Hazel Murphy, both physiotherapists at the Children's hospital. Hazel later emigrated to Australia with her husband and we still keep in touch. Father officiated at Sue's wedding and my parents came to know her parents, who were also supporters of the Royal National Lifeboat Institution. Liverpool friends and patients kept in touch; M (described earlier) had settled well with his new physiotherapist and later in the year was going to Sandfield Park Special school for handicapped children, which had a good reputation.

We had more snow during the winter of 1971 and realised that despite moving south the winters weren't any warmer. Thankfully we had Alfred and John the gardener to clear the long drives; the garages were 70 yards from the house and the road 200 yards from the garages. As we lived near bus routes, the roads were well gritted enabling me to get to work. At home we congregated in the large kitchen with its Aga stove.

Mother's ankle suffered a setback as she developed an ulcer under the plaster which required treatment for many months. However the bone healed and with my encouragement she exercised her ankle and regained full movement, enabling her to ride her bicycle to the local shops. She took a more active part in the diocese with Father and made friends locally. It was different from Liverpool as we lived next to the diocesan office with frequent official visitors, and Father was even busier than in Liverpool, with more responsibilities; he was often away from home.

He had the chauffeur Alfred to drive him round the diocese as the pressure of work was great and the roads a maze. We were told the city centre traffic had eased since building of the inner and outer ring roads, but you certainly needed to know exactly where you were going as dithering could be fatal. The Bullring was a landmark with its road system, and the covered market at a lower level attracted many shoppers. Alfred became a family friend and we corresponded at Christmas until his death. Since then I have kept in touch with one of his daughters.

Harborne was relatively peaceful although only three miles from the city centre and Bishop's Croft, surrounded by fields, very quiet. Even though Father was busy he delighted in hoisting St George's flag on the roof of the three storey red brick central block of the house on April 23rd, St George's day, Easter Day and Christmas Day.

Cousins called regularly, and Doris Kabity and Hazel, our friends from Liverpool, came to stay for

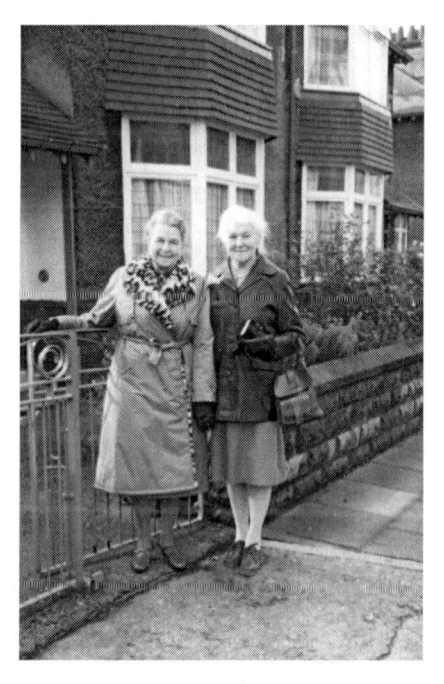

Mother with Doris Kabity, Auntie Doris, outside Doris' home in Liverpool

weekends and they enjoyed the house as much as Cupplesfield, and we explored the city together. Opposite the drive to the house was Grove Park, ideal for short walks with our dog, but as the weather improved we explored further and found a local golf course and the pleasant area around the Queen Elizabeth Hospital and University. Later we explored Ladywood reservoir and watched the sailing, and went further afield to the Lickey and Clent Hills which were easily accessible by car.

Petrena moved to Bishop's Croft at the end of March to start her new job at West Bromwich library, and regularly joined our weekend walks ; we explored Henley in Arden where we walked along the canal towpath and enjoyed its locally made ice creams; black cherry was my favourite. Although Petrena and I were again living at home we were by no means 'tied to our parents' apron strings' and had our own interests. My large bedsitting room had Hi-Fi equipment, sewing machine, and a desk for the typewriter. I had accepted that my days of playing squash were over so joined a badminton club with Petrena, but finding that it aggravated my wrist pain resigned after a couple of months.

Our family made St Peter's Church Harborne, just opposite the house, our parish church, though I joined Father on his diocesan visits to other churches on occasions. A service in Winson Green prison when Father licensed a new prison chaplain was my first experience of a prison: the grim atmosphere and clanging of the warden's huge bunches of keys impressed me. The prisoners regarded us with curiosity; most seemed sincere in their worship, singing lustily; staff said how much the chaplaincy was valued by them. By contrast a concert by the Royal Marine Band at the Town Hall was jolly and noisy.

As a diocesan bishop Father received an invitation in summer 1970 for himself, his wife and unmarried children to a garden party at Buckingham Palace. Alfred drove us into the Palace courtyard where we joined the queue going into the party. We walked through reception rooms with magnificent paintings and delicate china in highly polished antique cabinets. The gardens were colourful with rhododendrons and azalea as well as superb herbaceous borders. A band played jolly music and we joined other guests in official lines waiting for the Royal party who chatted to pre-selected guests; that year we saw the Queen and Duke of Edinburgh. Everyone was dressed for the occasion and Mother insisted I wear a hat, not my favourite item of clothing; Mother always wore one when she went out, having worked in the hat trade before she was married. Father had the choice of his purple episcopal cassock or gaiters and a frock coat, which he preferred, except that it was rather hot in summer; he didn't wear a hat. We met many of his fellow bishops and clerics and Caragh and Hugh Hanning with their son James, who I had looked after when he was a baby in the 1950s.

There were tables and chairs in front of the tea tents and those who had been there before advised us to get a table before we collected refreshments, as there were far more people than chairs. What a spread awaited us: delicate sandwiches, vol au vents, chocolate cakes and eclairs, strawberry tarts, and other fancy cakes. Never having tasted iced coffee, I thought it delicious and an excellent alternative to tea or cold drinks. Ice creams followed, which were much appreciated in the heat. Having heard about the pink flamingoes on the Palace lake we walked around the extensive grounds to see them, and it was hard to believe we were in central London and surrounded by busy roads just outside the Palace. Guests were expected to leave when the Royal party returned to the Palace, and Alfred was summoned over the loud speaker system.

Soon after the garden party my parents met Princess Anne when she visited Birmingham; they were favourably impressed.

In contrast, the following weekend Father and I went to a concert at Birmingham Town Hall, where Cliff Richard was the celebrity; he was a dedicated singer and we enjoyed the experience. In the autumn my parents were invited to a dinner party at 10 Downing Street by

Ted Heath, the Prime Minister; twenty years later, we met him in the Cathedral when he moved to a house in the Close in Salisbury.

I joined the Birmingham Festival Chorus, singing with them for the following five years until ill health forced me to resign, and Petrena played the flute with a small group. Sheila Whitehouse and Barbara and Derek Acock from the choir became particular friends. The latter lived very near Bishop's Croft, and we took their two young daughters Helene and Rosie to swim at the Queen Elizabeth Hospital pool. A nurse friend from work introduced me to the hospital leisure centre just five minutes from home; although never a keen swimmer I soon became a regular member of the pool, gradually gaining confidence and jumping into deep water. Elisabeth and Brian and the children also loved going there.

By Christmas 1970 we felt well settled and attended Birmingham Cathedral services and carol concerts which were more traditional than those at Liverpool. The Cathedral was an 18th-century parish church until the early 20th century when the Diocese was established.

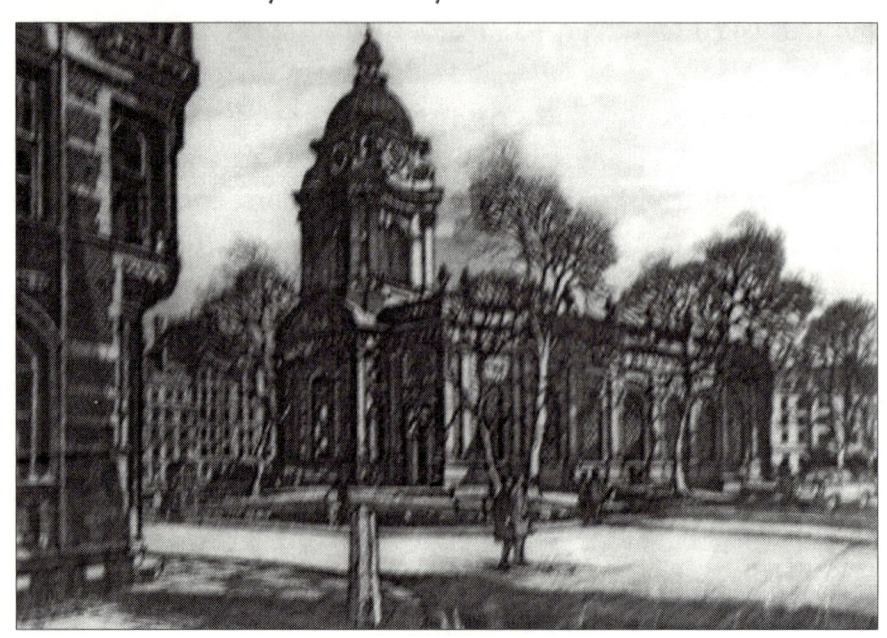

Sketch of Birmingham Cathedral

It is in the centre of the city among the business and shopping area and surrounded by a peaceful churchyard. It is much smaller and more intimate than Liverpool; several stunning Burne-Jones stained glass windows give colour to an otherwise grey building. After my father's death in 1994 a small memorial plaque was placed in the floor of the north side Chapel together with his prayer desk, inscribed with his name and the donors, the Vergers of Southwark Cathedral.

In 1971 Sheila, a new physiotherapist, and I enrolled for a genetics class, relevant to many patients who had inherited diseases. I sold my blue Fiat 500 to her and bought a new yellow/orange model which I called Golden Oxo; a couple of years later I had to change to an automatic car because of increasing health problems.

Our house was always busy with family, friends or official visitors and Mother often had to cater for large parties. Fortunately she had the offer of help from Iris Dickens, a parishioner in north-west Birmingham whom Father met when he preached at her church, who loved catering and brought her team with her. Functions were held at Bishop's Croft in the summer and Mother hosted a lively coffee morning every year for the Royal National Lifeboat Institution, raising several hundred pounds over the years. The kitchen at Bishop's Croft had an Aga and plenty of work surfaces, including four sinks in the kitchen, two in an adjoining butler's pantry, and another in the utility room.

Our home was a regular calling place for 'people of the road', as beggars liked to be called. Naturally they hoped we would be generous but we never gave money; instead we filled the often filthy tin jugs they carried with hot sweet tea, and offered them a sandwich or cake. If Father had discarded clothes we handed them over. The previous Bishop had helped them, so they said, and we were on their list of places to visit; they were polite and we came to recognise the regulars as they travelled round the country. Now living in a former chapel in Salisbury, I continue the practice of giving a mug of tea.

During the summer of 1971 when I was recovering from an elbow operation I had my first visit to the Birmingham Oratory where we listened to a performance of *The Dream of Gerontius*, with the choir of the Birmingham School of Music. This made a great impression on me particularly as the work was premiered at the Oratory in 1900.

Holidays

IN 1970 OUR first holiday was to a Liverpool friend's cottage in Anglesey, followed by a week at a clergy holiday house in Dunwich on the Suffolk coast. Anglesey was bleak even in July and the weather chilly throughout our stay; however on days when the sun shone Father and I bathed in the cold sea. The wild flowers were colourful and scenery spectacular with marvellous views along the coast of Wales. After a night at home we drove to Dunwich in Suffolk. The cottage was on the sea front and Father and I often bathed before breakfast; the water was considerably warmer. We visited Minsmere, a fascinating bird reserve newly developed since our holidays in the 1950s, also places like Walberswick and Blythburgh with its splendid Norman church, where we had been 20 years before. Elisabeth and Brian, when they moved to Walberswick some years later, worshipped at the latter church, and Elisabeth was later buried in the churchyard overlooking the river Blyth after her untimely death in 1995 from multiple sclerosis.

In spring 1971 I visited several friends near London, first spending a few days with Elisabeth and family at St Albans. We called on several old friends living nearby including Brown Owl, who had been leader of a Brownie pack which Elisabeth and Petrena joined in Welwyn Garden City where I was born. Afterwards we drove around old haunts known to me better by name than as places because we moved when I was five. In Luton we visited my godmother, Kathleen Weston, then I drove to Orpington in Kent to stay with Gladys Pichler, our former neighbour from Blackheath; I also met there Pat Lisle, a good friend from physiotherapy school days with her husband and two young boys. I had a day in Blackheath where I called on Caragh Hanning, and Mrs Henkel, our friend with whom we had spent Boxing Day each year. She had been seriously ill the year before but we were able to catch up with news of her husband, an excellent baker, and their children, Mary and Martin. The final day was spent at King's where my friend Margaret, whose accommodation I had taken over, still worked. She showed me the newly built physiotherapy school which was a great improvement on the old prefabricated buildings, and we met some tutors who were interested in my work, also my success in writing.

My parents and I returned to Pollensa in Majorca in early summer, joining Frank and Ethel Morris again at their villa. Flowers were plentiful and colourful and we relaxed by taking walks around the village and surrounding countryside. Our Spanish was improving and we managed to haggle over bargains in the local market. We drove to Palma where we visited the majestic and very ornate Cathedral; donkey carts lined up outside waited to take tourists around the city, but as many of the roads were cobbled we decided against.

Personal Health

A FEW WEEKS AFTER our move to Birmingham, I had to contact Dr Pearce, as colitis resulting from salmonella food poisoning the previous year still hadn't settled; he prescribed neutradonna.

In April as my right elbow continued to be painful, I went to see Mr Beddow at Whiston hospital, staying overnight with Doris and Hazel Kabity. Although the right wrist was improving blood tests showed continuing inflammation, so the elbow was injected with hydrocortisone which helped for a while. We also visited Miss Stewart, and M who was continuing to make progress.

When I saw Mr Beddow again he was concerned my elbows were becoming contracted (tightened) with adhesions around the insertions of the flexor muscles preventing full extension (straightening). He again injected cortisone into the elbow and prescribed stretching exercises.

As in Liverpool, particularly in winter, I seemed to catch germs from my patients, and sinusitis with severe nosebleeds required cauterisation. Fortunately the doctors at the Children's Hospital were happy to treat staff which saved time off.

The move from damp Liverpool hadn't helped my susceptibility to infections, and prolonged colitis made me tired. I managed a full day at work though found weekend duties, when we worked with minimum staff, exhausting. Patients in intensive care for example were extremely ill and needed treatment several times a day.

During the summer my general health was still unsatisfactory, with repeated attacks of diarrhoea and continued pain in my arms, plus an infected finger which eventually had to be lanced. I was referred to Dr Clifford Hawkins, a physician at Birmingham General Hospital, who arranged a barium swallow that showed my stomach was unusually slow to empty. Different drugs were to be tried to see which gave most improvement of the bouts of violent diarrhoea.

Thankfully in New Year 1971 we had additional staff which helped reduce the workload. However I had a succession of coughs and colds as well as painful joints and, whereas other members of staff recovered well, my general health remained poor. Lifting children and giving them chest percussion aggravated the pain, and when treating children with cerebral palsy, getting up from the floor caused pains in the back and legs. Mr Pearson, an orthopaedic surgeon at the General hospital thought local care would be better than travelling to Liverpool. He diagnosed 'golfer's elbow' in my right elbow and ordered electromyograms (tests on the electrical activity to and from the muscles and nerve endings). The tests were normal and he injected cortisone again. Swimming was encouraged.

The right elbow was operated on in May when adhesions (thickening) were removed. I again reacted badly to the anaesthetic and was off work for two and a half weeks. Now the left arm had become painful and I developed tingling in my left hand. At least strapping the right wrist helped.

Meanwhile I had seen Professor Anderson who continued to be concerned about my gastrointestinal hypersensitivity and allergy and prescribed large doses of vitamin C, but this didn't help.

In the autumn the District Physiotherapist, Miss Doreen Caney, at the Queen Elizabeth Hospital School of Physiotherapy arranged further investigations. I continued working to the best of my ability, and on what turned out to be my last working day at the Children's hospital, visited a special school for children with cerebral palsy at Kidderminster. The next morning I was seen by Mr Pearson who put me off work for at least two weeks. Two weeks became two months, and life would never be the same again.

10
My Career in the Balance ~ 1971-74

Personal Health

On Friday August 20th 1971, I was treating patients at the Children's Hospital, and the following Monday was myself off work, and welcomed by Wendy Beavis, the pleasant secretary who was later to become a close friend, before being treated by Miss Patrick, the Superintendent Physiotherapist at Birmingham General Hospital. There were two main treatment rooms, one for men and one for women, a large gymnasium, and a small room for individual treatments including ultraviolet therapy. After assessing my arm movements and strength, Miss Patrick gave me exercises to strengthen the arms and increase the range of movement in the right elbow which would not straighten fully since the operation. She treated this with ultrasound with slight improvement, but commented about my general lack of fitness and strength, surprising as I had worked and swum regularly. Because of persistent diarrhoea I was referred to Dr Peter Dykes, a consultant gastroenterologist at the General, who prescribed medicine for the colon, and put me off work for a further period. To build up endurance I was encouraged to increase the number of lengths swum in the pool, though diving irritated my back pain and was quickly banned. In addition I had to carry weights from one end of the gym to the other, climb up and down wall ladders, and aim a netball into a mock goalpost. The more I did the more tired

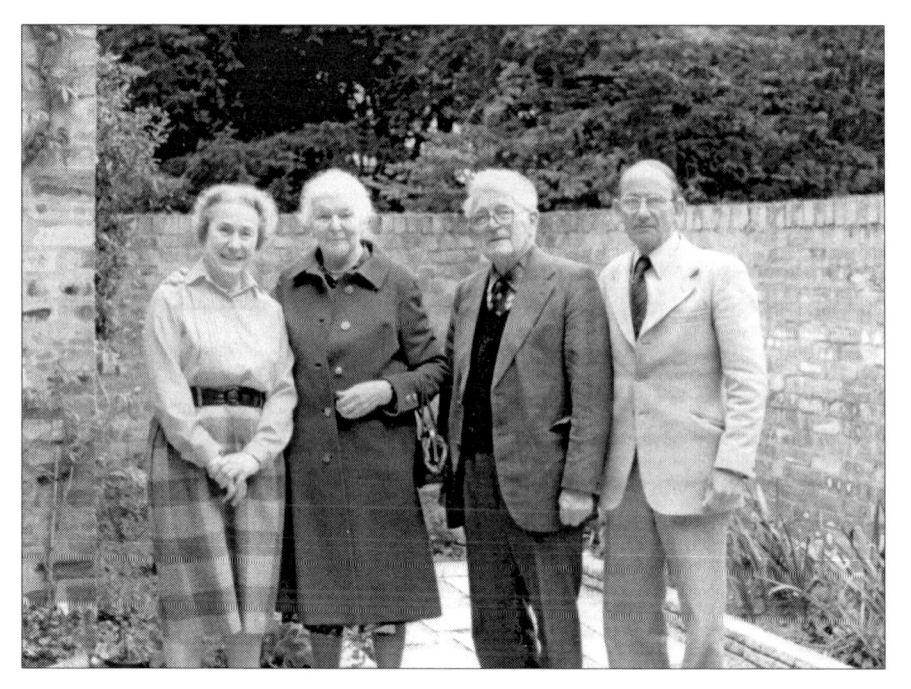

Wendy Beavis with my parents and a family friend

I became, and I began to worry about the long-term prospects for work.

After two months off sick, I was offered a three month trial at the General where there were more physiotherapists if I needed help, as a basic grade physiotherapist. The work aggravated the pain in my arms and back and was even more tiring than the therapy sessions but I didn't want to admit that work was too strenuous and when questioned tended to dissolve into tears. I saw Dr David Morgan, a psychiatrist at the Queen Elizabeth Hospital but he thought I was sensitive to atmosphere and to other peoples' moods and recommended continuing work.

Mr Pearson, Dr Dykes and Dr Morgan saw me regularly during the next three months but there was little improvement and I was becoming increasingly depressed.

In March 1972 I saw Professor Anderson at King's, who thought that as well as a hypersensitive gastrointestinal tract, I could have myasthenia gravis, a neurological disease in which there is a fault with transmission of chemicals between muscle and nerve endings resulting in fatigue which improves with rest. This seemed to fit my symptoms and although a lifelong condition, can be treated; and this improved my self-confidence.

During the next months my left thumb was very painful in addition to other joint and muscle pains. At first strapping was suggested, then ultrasound but a series of hydrocortisone injections into the joint were more helpful. Dr Dykes adjusted the medication for colitis several times, and having prescribed anti depressants Dr Morgan continued to see me at monthly intervals. In November the colitis became acute and I was put off work again. Maxalon to counteract the nausea and an opium derivative to calm the bowel didn't help. As my left arm was still painful a newer form of electrotherapy, microwave, produced some benefit. A new problem arose in the form of severe mouth ulcers and doctors at the Dental hospital recruited me to try out new treatments of tablets and creams they were developing.

Early in 1973 a biopsy of my small bowel was performed to exclude coeliac disease, a condition due to gluten sensitivity, but this proved inconclusive and other diagnoses such as mesenteric enteritis or bowel hypersensitivity were suggested.

In June 1973 I was admitted to King's. The weather was hot and sunny and when not needed for tests I could walk to nearby Ruskin Park or the physiotherapy department to see friends who worked there; as weekends were free I first went to Elisabeth in St Albans and then to Gladys Pichler at Orpington. I was seen by numerous different consultants and many blood tests and X rays were done, along with specialised investigations such as the tensilon test for myaesthenia, which proved inconclusive, and electromyograms (recording the electrical activity of the muscles) which were normal. A dietician provided special nourishing meals which other patients envied, and after a few days all tablets that had been prescribed in Birmingham were discontinued. After a week, hydrotherapy (physiotherapist supervised exercises in a heated pool) started and I was given specific exercises to strengthen my back muscles.

Many friends visited including Gladys Pichler, Sue Wilson who was Elisabeth's best friend from Blackheath High School, Peter Pichler and his wife Margaret, and Pat Lisle, my physiotherapy friend. My parents and Wendy Beavis, the secretary at the General, also came and kept me up to date with home life.

After two weeks Professor Anderson gave the results of the tests: the muscles and nerves were normal but the control of muscles was at fault. The cause was unknown but he hoped treatment with pyridostigmine bromide (which is also used to treat myaesthenia) would help, together with other tablets to treat my stomach problems, and a back support. He advised me to give up work as a physiotherapist because it was too strenuous for my weakened muscles, and suggested alternatives such as clinical supervisor for physiotherapy, technician for testing the heart or brain activity, dietician, medical secretary or work at the university.

Back home and off work I swam, rested when tired and walked our new dog, Suki. After Judy's death we had all missed having a dog and tried the local RSPCA first, but with no success, so went to an animal sanctuary where there were goats, some with three legs, rabbits, cats, chickens and dogs in a rather downbeat, small farm. A very scruffy, rough haired terrier held my attention. She was in a wooden box with other larger dogs but when she peeped out of the box and looked at me with her big brown eyes I felt she needed us. She was about eight months old and we christened her Suki; she remained with us as a friend and companion till her death in Salisbury in 1985.

Visits to other hospital and university departments about possible work took time and energy but after seeing the electroencephalography (EEG), and electromyography (EMG), cancer registry, X ray and numerous other departments, the only possibility seemed medical secretarial work. I needed shorthand and typing skills so signed on at nearby Selly Oak evening institute for the following term.

I changed my car to a DAF with automatic transmission to make driving easier; the fact that it had rubber bands for the transmission was a source of amusement.

After two months off I decided to return to physiotherapy, the job I enjoyed. At first I worked till mid-day, then gradually increased to nearly full time. The dose of pyridostigmine was increased which certainly helped muscle function, but indomethacin for the pain caused nausea and a recurrence of the colitis, even with suppositories. My eyes then became swollen and this was thought to be an allergic reaction. All tablets were stopped and cortisone cream prescribed, which proved effective. After a 'patch test' when different plant samples were taped to my back, an allergy to nickel and the geranium plant family were suggested as the cause of my swollen eyes.

I was doing well with the touch typing and pitmanscript course despite the arm pain; an electric typewriter helped because it required less pressure, though handwriting was difficult as cramp affected my right hand and limited the speed I could take dictation.

The following three months were very difficult. Work certainly aggravated the pains in my arms and back and I became exhausted more quickly. Many different drugs were tried including phenylbutazone which caused an irritating rash, Primalgen and amitriptlyne with little benefit and adverse side effects.

Furthermore there was disagreement amongst the doctors and they decided I would be treated in Birmingham by Dr Dykes and not by Professor Anderson in London. Eventually I was sent home feeling sick and very weak with acute colitis, and on April 24th 1974 I was signed off work; my last day working as a physiotherapist, the career I had chosen and enjoyed for eleven years.

✶ *My Career in the Balance* ✶

Work 1971-1974

In September 1971, although off sick, I attended an interesting course on paediatric physiotherapy at Guy's Hospital London, not knowing I wouldn't be able to return to work with children. Even though working with adults was very different, it was good to go back. There was far more instruction to adult patients, and we regularly used machines in treatments, such as shortwave diathermy for deep heat treatment, infra-red for more superficial heat, ultra-violet light therapy for skin conditions, and ultrasound for pain and inflammation.

Junior staff worked on a rota system, treating patients on the wards, the outpatient department, gym or a small room for varying forms of light therapy. My first three months were spent on the wards, then moving on to outpatients where I was in charge of the women's department for a few days, so felt my work must be satisfactory. Soon after I was assured the post was long term so with experience there might be a vacant senior post. I still felt out of place because I was older and had more experience, as well as having supervised several of the juniors at the Children's hospital.

I was asked to take over the men's orthopaedic ward with help from a student and all went smoothly. We had two contrasting types of patients: the young and fit with a sporting injury and elderly patients in need of joint, usually hip, replacement, sometimes after a fall, often unfit and needing specific exercises before being mobilised with crutches or walking frames. They were often heavy and needed two or three people to assist. When the senior post was advertised I applied, but a young friend, whom I had supervised as a student, was appointed.

My next move was to in-patient relief work including the intensive care unit, and then general relief where I stayed to the end of my working days at the General. When any member of staff was on leave or off sick I looked after their patients, certainly good for adaptability, both physically and mentally, but I felt like a spare part and less secure than ever. There seemed no way I could return to work in paediatrics; adult work, though less physical than paediatrics, still exacerbated pain in my back and arms, and made me very tired.

An encounter in early 1974 had long term consequences. I was working in the women's outpatient department and a child of eleven called Karen appeared for treatment at 8.30am. As the senior physiotherapist was often occupied at that time, she would organise Karen's treatment, and then instruct me to supervise and send her off to school. Karen had an undiagnosed pain and lack of function in her right wrist. Various treatments had been tried without success, and it was suggested that she might be suffering from a psychosomatic disorder. I tried treating her with wax baths and encouraging wrist and finger movements by playing table games (which I took in from

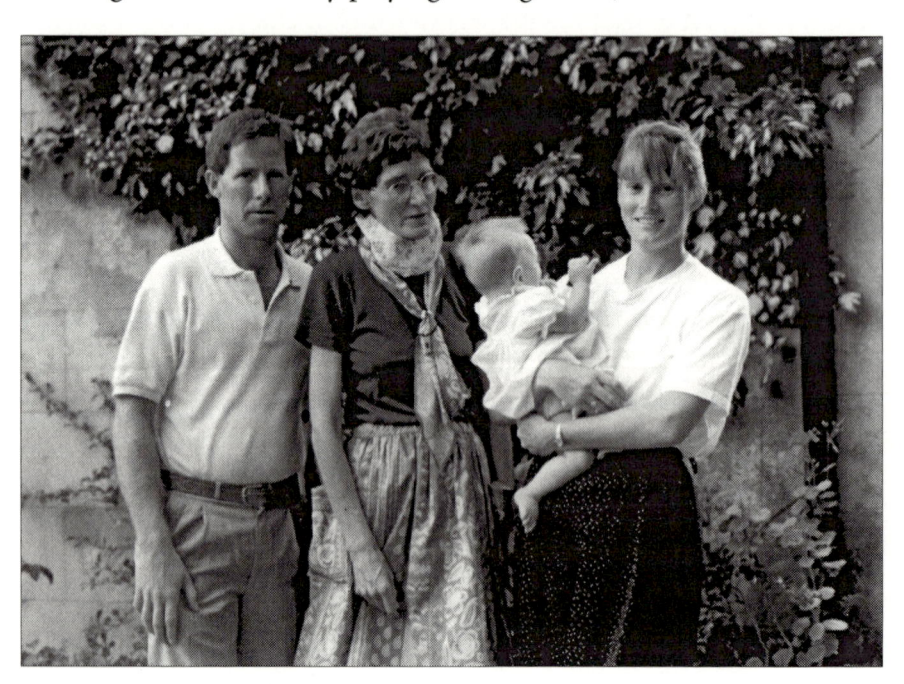

Karen and Anthony Hathaway with their first child, Laura.

home), as we did not have such equipment in the Department. She was soon cured and asked if she could remain in touch when discharged. I didn't expect to hear from her, but a few months later after I finished work at the General, she started visiting me at home. In due course she qualified as a nurse and is now happily married with two children and we meet up whenever possible.

Wax baths were used particularly for the treatment of hands and feet. Medical wax was heated in a suitably lined container to a certain temperature; the affected part was then immersed several times, allowing each coating to dry before the next immersion. After the final coat had dried the hand (or foot) was wrapped in greaseproof paper with towels on top to maintain the heat for a few minutes. The wax was then peeled off, leaving it warm and hopefully more mobile.

In November 1972 I was offered the post of senior physiotherapist in sole charge at the geriatric hospital in East Birmingham. After much thought I declined because geriatric work is heavy and involves physical work which I hadn't the strength to do.

Holidays

My first holiday during these difficult years was to visit friends in and around London. I stayed with Margaret Jenkinson in Herne Hill and while there visited Professor Anderson and friends at King's. Next I drove to Orpington, passing through old haunts of Greenwich Park and the water front; Gladys Pichler was always welcoming and while there Pat Lisle née Dee and I met up. The following day Petrena and I met at Welwyn Garden City Hospital where she had a job interview. I took the opportunity to visit the physiotherapy department and was impressed to see physiotherapists working closely with occupational therapists, which I missed at the General. We returned home calling on Elisabeth at St Alban's, never missing an opportunity to see her when in the area.

In June 1972, despite not feeling well I went to Scotland again to stay with Auth Ruth's sister, Joyce and her family who had moved to Edinburgh. James and Joyce Rogers were busy people, and the children at school, so I spent the days with my guidebook using the local bus and train service, as the house was in the suburbs. I visited Holyrood Palace, Carlton Hill, with its view of St Mary's Cathedral, Edinburgh Castle, the Camera Obscura, the Museum of Childhood, and Greyfriars. Joyce also took me to the local market and I visited several of the City's art galleries. I took the train to the Forth Bridge, but as it was a wet June day didn't enjoy the full splendour of that vast metal structure, and explored the coast by train to North Berwick, which was then a small village on the widening river.

Later that year Petrena and I had a week's holiday in north Wales, an area we didn't know. A friend of Father's invited us to use his cottage in the small village of Pont Fadog. The weather was good and every day we went out visiting Chirk, Llangollen, Corwen, Bala, Oswestry, Sellatyn and Llanrhaiadr waterfalls. The wooded areas were attractive with early morning mists and the leaves changing colour. Blackberries were easy to find and we picked some to eat most days; they always seem to taste better off the hedges.

In 1973 I visited Ann and Barry Davies in Barnack. Their children, Richard and Rachel, aged about 4 and 5 years old were again delighted to show me the 'hills and holes', an area of uneven ground near their home resulting from quarrying of the local Stamford stone some years previously. Ann and Barry took me to Stamford, where Barry taught at the old Grammar School, Peterborough with its magnificent Cathedral, and their own village of Barnack.

In March Petrena and I returned to north Wales, not knowing that this would be our last holiday together. We were able to go back to favourite places and explore more of North Wales. We also went to Liverpool to see the Anglican Cathedral (which had been extended further west since we left the city) and to visit Doris and Hazel Kabity, as well as my former patients, Miss Stewart and M.

✳ *My Career in the Balance* ✳

In July I returned to Swan Lake cottage with my parents for a few days relaxation, returning home via Poole where Father preached at a Boy Scout Service on Brownsea Island. Mother and I enjoyed the boat trip over to the island and found the service moving with hundreds of Scouts from the area singing hymns lustily in the open air chapel. We returned home via Salisbury, where we would come to live some years later.

My last holiday that year was to Sedbergh, Cumbria where Auntie Margaret and I stayed a few days with cousin Jenny and her husband Robin Hildrew who was a teacher at the boys' public school. The journey was memorable for I had just taken delivery of the second-hand DAF, which turned out to be rather unreliable. The oil light lit but the AA couldn't find the fault, then the front shelf fell off, dropping maps and other papers on to our feet. Despite the car problems we had a wonderful time walking along Winder Fell with superb views of the countryside, visiting Kendal and the Abbot Hall Museum and church. Another day we took a ferry to Sawry, the home of Beatrix Potter, returning via Hawkshead. We went to Sedbergh market, then to Hawes and Cotter Force to see the noisy waterfall. That day we returned home via Buttertubs where we had fantastic views of the surrounding countryside over the moors and fells and Hardsaw Fall. We had to return home earlier than expected as Uncle Roland became acutely ill and Aunt Margaret had to travel to Dorchester to help Aunt Ruth nurse him.

Social Life

After my therapy sessions at Birmingham General in 1971 when I was off work, I explored parts of the city previously unknown to me. As so often happens when you live in a place visitors seem to explore more than locals. I found the canal and canal basin, which since we moved have been improved beyond recognition, the jewellery quarter near St Paul's Church and the back streets of the city. I had more time to enjoy the Art Gallery and Museum and my local knowledge greatly increased.

At home, Tony and Madeline Stroud from Salisbury and Mrs Doris Kabity and Hazel from Liverpool were regular visitors to Bishop's Croft. Auntie Margaret's best friend, Miss Freda Critchley, also visited. I continued to keep in touch by letter with many friends, from my schooldays, at King's College Hospital, and from Liverpool.

When attending a paediatric course at Guy's I stayed with Margaret Jenkinson, a friend from King's. She took me to the vast Crystal Palace Sports Centre to watch an athletics event and have a swim in their Olympic size pool. On my return journey I stayed with Elisabeth and enjoyed sharing my goddaughter Rachel's birthday outing to Whipsnade Zoo.

At home, Barbara Acock whom I had met at the Birmingham Festival Choral Society, started to come swimming and we regularly took her two young daughters Helene and Rose, who quickly gained confidence in the water. They lived very near Bishop's Croft and have remained friends for the last thirty-five years. Father started regular swimming too which pleased Mother; he needed exercise and relaxation as his work was very demanding.

When Father, as Bishop of Birmingham, set off with Mother to visit the link diocese of Malawi, Petrena, Auntie Margaret and I took charge of the house and Judy, our dog. Petrena was working at Solihull library but I was off work so could sort Father's post and deliver the official mail to his secretary at Church House. The conditions in Malawi in 1971 were very primitive with poor housing and low incomes; my parents' experiences included being given a live chicken as they left a settlement, and flying in a tiny open aircraft to get to the dedication of a new cathedral on an island on Lake Malawi. They found the people very welcoming and enthusiastic about their faith, and had many happy memories of the visit.

Christmas 1971 was enjoyable. After the services in Birmingham we went to St Albans to share the excitement with Elisabeth and family. They lived near the Abbey and Verulamium (the Roman remains of the old town) which were familiar to my parents who had grown up in nearby Luton. In the New Year Petrena became a volunteer helper at Birmingham Maternity hospital shop and often asked me to help; we enjoyed being shop assistants selling such things as baby clothes and toys. I also started playing the piano regularly, hoping it would strengthen my wrists, and after a couple of months decided to have professional lessons with Mrs Hazlehurst, a teacher at the Birmingham School of Music, whose first comment was that my fingers needed strengthening.

Wendy Beavis came swimming regularly and often returned to Bishop's Croft afterwards for a meal. Later we took up ballroom dancing. As our friendship developed we went for weekend walks exploring further afield in Warwickshire and Worcestershire to such places as Stratford-upon-Avon and small villages, taking a picnic so we could relax and enjoy a chat wherever we wanted. Wendy lived with her parents in Four Oaks, North Birmingham and sometimes I drove over and we went north exploring Lichfield and its Cathedral, the Derby Dales and the villages. As we both enjoyed music we went to concerts at the Town Hall, the Cathedral and the Barber Institute to hear various orchestras including the City of Birmingham Symphony Orchestra. In this way we heard John Lill and Yehudi Menuhin giving stunning recitals. Later we went on holidays to stay with my family friend, Biddy Carrick, who lived at Stratton near Bude in North Cornwall. After we moved I kept in touch with Wendy by correspondence and she visited us in Salisbury occasionally until her death a few years later.

Other visitors to our house were Angela and Tony Lambert, who I had met at the squash club in Great Crosby. Since returning from their round-the-world trip following their wedding, they eventually settled in Devon in the picturesque village of Branscombe. Angela's mother lived at Alcester, south of Birmingham, and Angela often visited us when staying there. We went swimming in the brine baths at

Droitwich, an interesting experience floating like a cork in the warm salty water. The baths were in the original 18th-century building and small changing rooms surrounded the water with wooden steps down into the bath. Part of the enjoyment was getting out when an attendant enveloped each swimmer with a very large heated towel. I don't know if it did any good, but it was certainly fun. Angela worked as an art teacher at local schools while Tony trained as a mature student to become a very successful language teacher. They had two children, Jamie and Tessa, and I had several happy holidays with them at their cottage, aptly called Brookside, because of a bubbling stream passing through the garden.

Every year my parents and I went to a garden party at Buckingham Palace. We met friends and enjoyed the atmosphere, and after Father's retirement as diocesan bishop were invited every three years and accepted until Mother's health made social outings difficult. After a wonderful holiday in Kenya visiting friends, Uncle Roland, Father's brother, became ill with leukaemia in autumn 1972. Once stabilised he continued living a busy life, involved with music events and Scottish dancing at his home in Dorchester until his death in 1976.

I decided to take a short course in candle making at a local evening institute and made sufficient candles to decorate the house and give to friends for Christmas 1972. The Aga helped to heat the wax and Mother tolerated having rows of dripping candles hanging from kitchen cupboard knobs; by immersing a wick in heated wax, then leaving it hanging to dry before repeating the process, the candle gradually thickened, and colours can be added to the wax.

In April 1973, after Petrena and I had a week's holiday in North Wales, she and Michael Camps announced their engagement. They planned to marry in the autumn and were busy house hunting, eventually buying a house in Yardley Wood. Mother organised the reception which was to be at Bishop's Croft, with Iris Dickens and her team making the cake and refreshments. Auntie Margaret was busy *(above) Jenny and Robin Hildrew on their wedding day. (left) Petrena and Michael Camps on their wedding day outside Bishop's Croft*

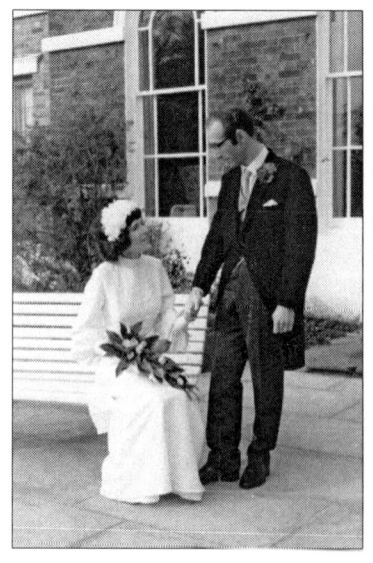

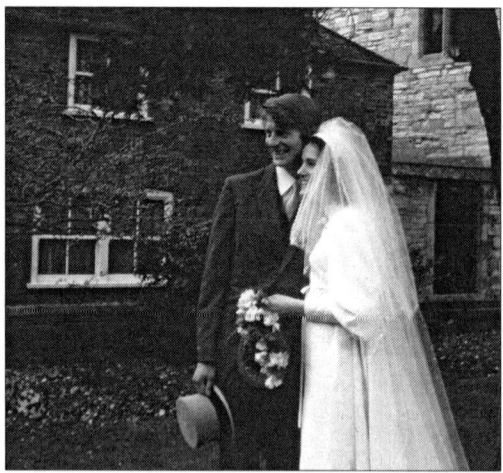

making bridesmaids' dresses for my nieces, Sarah and Rachel, and I had to buy a suitable outfit. The day of the wedding was sunny and mellow and we all walked to St Peter's Church, Harborne, just five minutes from Bishop's Croft. The guests returned to the house and the party went on all evening. We had a full house with Elisabeth and family, Uncle Roland, Aunt Ruth and cousin Sue staying, also Doris and Hazel Kabity from Liverpool.

Earlier in the year my cousin Jenny Brown married Robin Hildew, a long time friend from when both families lived at Grasmere. Father performed the wedding at Dorchester and we spent the weekend at Swan Lake cottage which was within easy reach. Uncle Roland and Aunt Ruth gave an excellent party at their house after the wedding; they had a billiard room which was ideally suited to the tradition of a Scottish dancing party. The following day Father christened cousin Chris Brown's first baby, Rachel. It was good having all the family together and Uncle Roland, despite his illness, was able to enjoy the double celebration.

A few weekends later Wendy and I went to hear a performance of the *The Magic Flute* by Mozart and this changed my life: I decided

※ *Walking on Wheels* ※

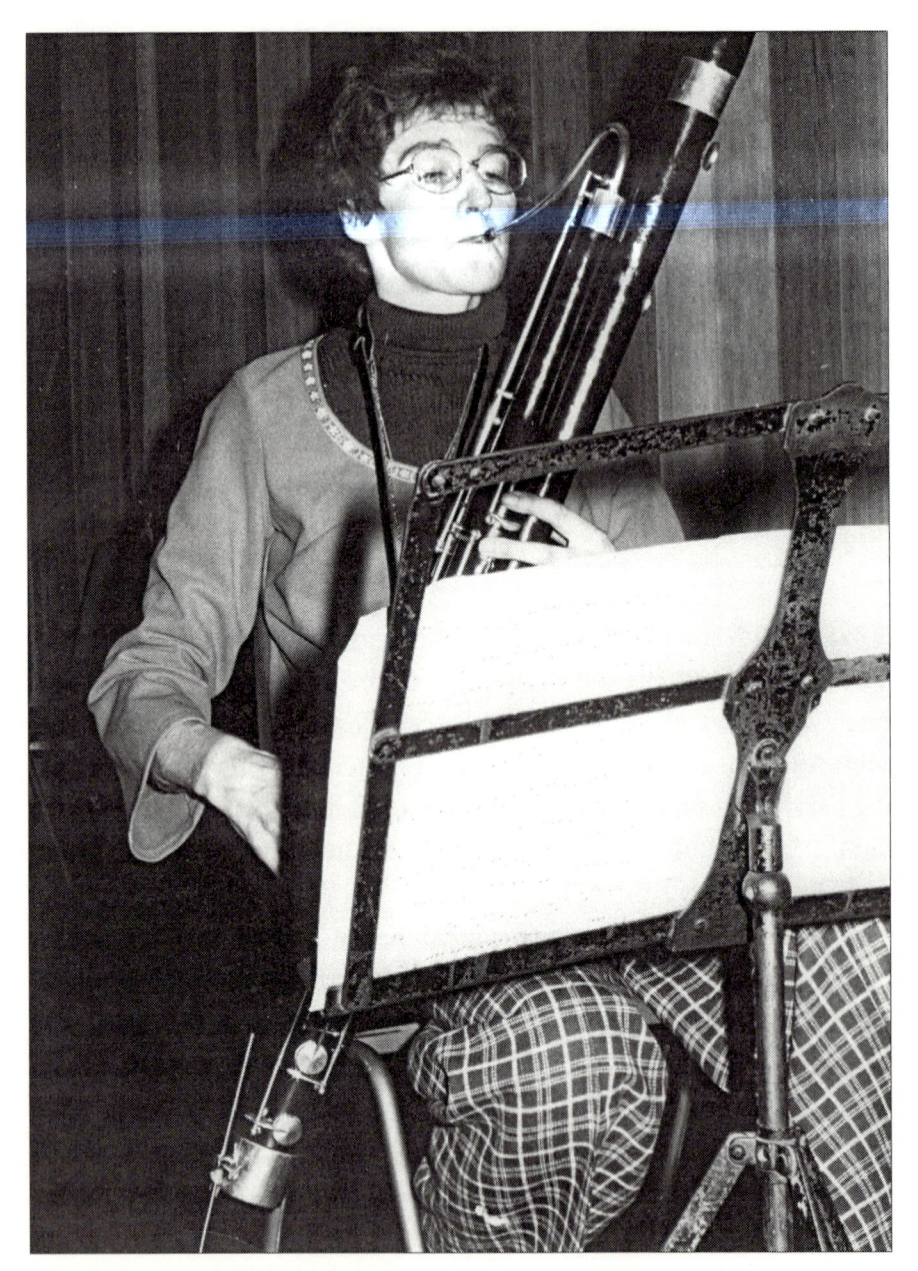

Jill playing her bassoon in Birmingham

to take up playing a wind instrument to enable me to join an amateur orchestra. Friends advised there were too many clarinet and flute players, so an oboe or bassoon was suggested. Mrs Cowsill, a woodwind teacher brought a bassoon for me to try, as an oboe required a great deal of puff. She was amazed, when on my first attempt I played a note and the mellow sound appealed so I decided to learn to play. I was able to buy a bassoon from a lad called Jonathan, a pupil of Mrs Cowsill, who spent time teaching me so that I could play a simple tune by the time of my first lesson. I nicknamed the instrument 'Bertie' and 'he' gave me great pleasure for the next few years. I also resumed piano lessons with Frank Wibaut who had taken over when Mrs Hazlehurst retired, and who also taught at the Birmingham School of Music. This was the start of another friendship, and later he asked me to do some secretarial work for him.

Evening classes, bassoon and piano lessons, and necessary swimming, in addition to work, were tiring and I had to restrict other social life. I resigned from the Birmingham Festival Choral Society.

Father, who as a senior bishop took turns in saying prayers at the House of Lords before a sitting, gave us lunch at the members dining room of the House. It was gracious and old fashioned, and I was overwhelmed by the courtesy and formality. We walked along dark corridors with lush décor, and even found the toilets elegant and comfortable.

When Margaret Jenkinson from London came to stay for a weekend we went to the Walsgrave Hospital in Coventry for a demonstration of a revolutionary innovation for disabled people, a Possum machine. This could be adapted to suit each person's needs, for example by operating equipment such as lighting, telephone, TV, radio and electric typewriters and unlocking and locking doors; it was controlled by easy-to-use electronic switches. This was a revolutionary life-line in the early 1970s for those who were partially paralysed or otherwise incapacitated and we were very impressed at how much independence it would give to many of our patients. I joined the Possum Users Association as a life member not knowing that I myself would need such equipment later.

11
Confusion
May 1974 – June 76

When I recovered from the acute bout of colitis in May, my first thoughts were to find another less physical job. I made an appointment at the Professional Advisory bureau to see Miss Tilley the disability officer, but my medical problem needed to be identified before she could help.

Personal Health

After a week's holiday with Wendy Beavis in Cornwall I saw Dr Dykes, and was signed off work to give up physiotherapy for the time being: Miss Caney, Principal of the Physiotherapy School at the Queen Elizabeth Medical Centre reminded me that 'when the Lord closes one door He always opens other windows'. This has proved true throughout my illness and I remind myself of that at difficult times.

Earlier in May I had an appointment with Dr Michael Small, neurologist. He ordered special blood tests, a muscle biopsy and electromyograms (electrical tests) on my muscles and referred me to Mrs Jenny Lee, a social worker, who was to be a great strength to me during the following years, talking over problems and liasing between doctors and staff at the rehabilitation unit where I was later sent. She gave up work after her son was born in 1975 but we remain friends.

Confusion

The electromyograms and muscle biopsies in June were done at the Queen Elizabeth Medical Centre in Edgbaston. These proved inconclusive, however repeat tests three months later (in October) showed inflammatory changes in the muscles and abnormal electromyograms indicating myositis. CorticoSteroids (prednisone) were prescribed with other drugs. Over the summer months of 1974 Dr Dykes organised an insulin tolerance test to check the function of my pituitary gland (which regulates the proper activity of other endocrine glands) but again the results were unhelpful, and psychological factors were suggested although Dr Morgan, psychiatrist, had discharged me nine months earlier.

The health visitor at our surgery was very supportive and saw me at regular intervals to check my general health. Meanwhile in June Mr Harrison (orthopaedic surgeon) operated on my right wrist and found a tight retinaculum (band of fibres); this certainly accounted for the pain I had experienced. In August he operated on the left wrist and found a similar tightness, which was also removed with similar good results. He suggested finding a job but after a necessary medical at the local Department of Health and Social work I was declared unfit to work and referred to the disabled resettlement officer (DRO) who registered me as disabled: that seemed very final and I was dismayed.

In September 1974 Mrs Lee suggested I have an assessment for fitness to work at the Industrial Rehabilitation Unit at Edgbaston (IRU). I was interviewed by Mr Brennan in charge of the IRU, to decide if I was suitable for the scheme and I was accepted. The unit had different departments such as office work, light engineering and heavy engineering, to assess candidates' capability and fitness for work. At first I went for half days and was put to work copying script by hand. This caused cramps like I had experienced at pitmanscript classes so I was sent to the light workshop where I assembled plugs; this was very easy but tedious. Soldering was attempted but exacerbated the pain in my wrists, so I was put on switchboard work in the office to rest my wrists. The newly opened unit was publicized on local television at the time and I was shown working, much to my friends' amusement.

After ten days I attended for two thirds of the day which left me too exhausted to go to the pool afterwards to do my exercises. Wrist pain was also aggravated so splints were made to measure at the General Hospital. I was encouraged to continue despite the fatigue and usually had to lie down and rest in the sick bay at lunch time. Even then I was regularly sent home early, so a three day week was suggested. The light workshop where I used electronic calculators for maths and did typing was more suitable, though endurance was still a problem. There I met a volunteer social worker, Mrs Ruth Wolfe, who suggested an electric typewriter would be easier physically and she later arranged for me to have one for use at home.

By December any progress had been limited by poor endurance and muscle strength. A few weeks after taking prednisone, phlebitis (inflammation of a vein) in my right leg was suspected: I was to rest and not return to the rehabilitation unit. I was disappointed as this was to be the route to finding a suitable job.

By Christmas Miss Caney suggested I apply for a retirement pension as it seemed unlikely my health would improve sufficiently for me to return to an active job like physiotherapy.

My health was not improving and the following month the dose of prednisone was increased several times. I developed a urinary tract infection, nausea and then swollen legs and prednisone was reduced. I was referred to Professor Walton, consultant neurologist, for admission to the specialist Neuromuscular Centre at Newcastle upon Tyne. The electromyograms were repeated and at last there was some improvement in muscle function, though my general health continued to deteriorate, with weight loss and a rapid pulse; a fall on my knee didn't help.

Archdeacon Harry Bates, our former vicar in Crosby then in Newcastle, met me at the station and took me to hospital. He and his wife visited me, as did Jane Scott, a physiotherapist I worked with

✳ Confusion ✳

at Birmingham who had moved north, the hospital chaplain and a friend of Archdeacon Bates, Mrs Dorothy Chapman. We became friends and corresponded until her death.

A team of neurologists including Dr Hudson and Dr Foster saw me as well as Professor Walton and many tests including electromyograms, electrocardiograms, X rays of my arms and back, and blood tests were taken. A urinary infection was again diagnosed for which antibiotics were prescribed. The dose of prednisone was reduced and medication for colitis was prescribed. The diagnosis was steroid myopathy (muscle wasting) which should recover as the dose of steroid was gradually withdrawn.

After ten days I returned home and continued reducing the prednisone gradually. I was advised to be as active as possible within the limits of pain and exercise tolerance, and to reduce wearing the back support over the coming months. Valium tablets had been prescribed but these were discontinued after three weeks because they didn't help and side effects were untoward.

As arranged I returned to Newcastle in July 1975; although the electromygrams had returned to normal, my muscle power and exercise tolerance hadn't improved as much as Professor Walton had anticipated. I was still underweight, with undiagnosed digestive problems, muscle wasting and muscle fatigue. I had been prescribed amitriptyline but these were stopped after less than a week because of adverse side effects; I felt 'spaced out' and reversed my car into the front of Father's official car causing considerable damage to the bonnet, and further reducing my self confidence. I also fell over again and cut my leg so badly I needed regular dressings and tetanus injections from the district nurse for a few weeks. An alternative medication, imipramine, was prescribed but this was stopped after two weeks because of confusion; substitution of prothiaden affected eye focusing so was also discontinued.

I was determined to attempt working and started a few hours' office work, first at Church House for Father's colleagues covering for holiday absences, then, after an interview at the Queen Elizabeth Hospital relief audio typing and general office work in various departments. I could manage only a few hours at a time because of inability to sit unsupported holding my arms in a typing position. Holding a pen for shorthand was restricted too so audio typing was preferable, but I enjoyed meeting people and being out working, and continued while there was a job. Later, staff from the department of Mechanical Engineering at the University gave me work to type at home, though terminology was often a puzzle. Mrs Christine King, occupational therapist, had supplied me with a high-backed armchair, which enabled me to type longer. Later Frank Wibaut, my piano teacher, gave me work.

Voluntary work included reading for the Royal National Institute for the Blind who had a centre near Harborne. They supplied me with books or periodicals requested by local blind people which needed transferring on to tape. A regular task was to read the monthly physiotherapy journal for a blind physiotherapist, and a long-term project was to record the Be-Ro cookery book. As my respiratory muscles were becoming affected, I was only able to record for a limited time.

There was no real improvement in my health during 1975, trials of different drugs were unhelpful, and the doctors couldn't agree what the problem was.

Mrs King continued to visit and together we went to pottery classes at Canon Hill Art Centre. We hoped moulding clay would strengthen my wrists and arms and work on a wheel would strengthen my back; we both enjoyed the sessions. I had found that resting between periods of activity enabled me to continue for longer periods and during the term made several pots and dishes which we used at home.

The year 1976 brought a change in understanding of my medical condition. Mr Harrison decided not to operate further on my arms for three months and suggested the pain could be from nerve roots in the neck, so posture was important. More eye cysts were removed at the Queen Elizabeth Hospital. The colitis was still severe: a fat free diet was suggested and at last there was some improvement in my digestion and the colitis. I had been making and eating a lot of yoghurt and milk puddings, so changed to a milk free diet, in addition to fat free, with further benefit.

Father asked a colleague from a medical religious advisory committee, Dr George Hearn, to see me; Dr Hearn had a special interest in chest disease and food allergy. He was certain my digestive problems were caused by food allergy and advised following a gluten and milk free diet and avoiding other foods that aggravated the colitis.

A few weeks later Dr Pearce referred me back to Professor John Anderson at King's. I was to be admitted as soon as a bed was available. In July 1976 I returned to King's and stayed for five months.

Social Life

SOCIAL LIFE WAS restricted by my health but I learnt that taking rests between activities enabled me to do more. I continued making music, having bassoon lessons with Mrs Cowsill, and soon friends accompanied me on the piano. I then joined the WEA (Workers Educational Association) orchestra at nearby Ladywood. The conductor, Anthony Millar, welcomed me, bassoon players being in short supply, and other members collected me from home when driving became a problem. After some months several woodwind players, including Joy Williamson, suggested we play together as a sextet or octet, meeting at Bishop's Croft, where the first floor landing was ideal and the sound radiated around the house which the family enjoyed. Joy and I still correspond and exchange news about families and musical activities. After some months I was invited to play with the Canon Hill orchestra as well, and when my lungs weakened the conductor agreed I play as many notes as I could providing the main bass notes.

Swimming was encouraged as part of my treatment and I went to the pool at Queen Elizabeth hospital regularly, and was often joined by friends. The Saturday morning swimming club for handicapped children, hearing of my past paediatric physiotherapy experience, requested help. I was in my element assisting with the children and the buoyancy of the water supported both their body weight and mine making movement easier, but after a few months I wasn't able to continue as my health deteriorated. As a challenge I attempted the Amateur Swimming Association badges, summating the number of lengths swum over a period until reaching bronze, then silver and finally gold. There was no time limit so I added as many lengths as I felt able at each session and eventually achieved gold. Another regular swimmer was Georgina Thompson (née) Shentall, an orthoptist at the hospital with whom I have kept in touch. She now visits me in Salisbury from her home near Southampton.

We had numerous visitors to Bishop's Croft: Elisabeth with her family, Doris and Hazel Kabity and Daisy and Fred stayed regularly. We saw Petrena and Michael most weeks either at Bishop's Croft or at their home in south Birmingham. Julia, Professor Anderson's secretary, had become a friend and visited us from South London; on one occasion we went to a fair at Canon Hill Park where she was much more adventurous than me, enjoying attractions that I was happier to watch.

Elisabeth had introduced me to Ilsa and Joe Heaton and their young family of three boys who had moved to Edgbaston from Stockton on Tees where they were near neighbours of hers. We went swimming, and walking in the Lickey or Clent Hills and Ilsa and I went to concerts, including the Verdi *Requiem* at the City Hall. Concerts became something of a problem when sitting on hard chairs at the City Hall with no support for my neck, so I bought a portable car headrest which fitted on the back of the seat and together with a cushion eased the situation.

My parents were increasingly busy and entertained several overseas visitors to the diocese, some staying at Bishop's Croft. Sir

Arthur Chetwynd from Toronto in Canada had links through his family with a small parish and school in the north of the diocese, and on the first visit with his wife, Marjorie, met my parents. Subsequently when they came to Birmingham they stayed with us at Bishop's Croft and later came to Salisbury when Father had retired. My parents stayed with them in 1975 when they were invited to spend five weeks in Canada, Father preaching at their Church, St Paul's in Toronto. While they were in Canada I stayed with the Strouds in their Salisbury home and explored the city as well as visiting Swan Lake cottage. We discussed Father's retirement, in November 1977, when he would be 70. It was they who suggested we move to Salisbury and Tony found a small former chapel within walking distance of the Cathedral, which has remained my home to the present day.

HRH Princess Margaret came to Birmingham for a busy schedule of official engagements, including opening a parish hall, and rested at Bishop's Croft before the ceremony.

Wendy Beavis was a good friend and we usually met for swimming after her day's work at the General. We had both passed the typing and pitmanscript exams and she had been promoted from receptionist to secretary. When my parents were away she stayed the night, as they were loathe to leave me alone in the large secluded house. At weekends we took Suki with us to explore the countryside around Birmingham, the Malvern Hills, Stratford-on-Avon and Lapworth along the canal bank, all favourite summer walks.

Holidays

WENDY AND I joined my parents at Swan Lake cottage for a short visit to Dorset in 1974. Aunt Ruth and Uncle Roland had joined us for a picnic along with members of the Stroud family and we all picked strawberries for our meal from a local fruit farm as well as enjoying the lake and it surrounds. At the time there was great excitement about Zeffirelli's film *Jesus of Nazareth*: my parents had been invited at short notice to represent the Church of England in Rome for its première. All expenses including flights and accommodation at a first class hotel would be paid. Fortunately the message didn't arrive until the day of our return and we had enjoyed a good weekend. My parents thoroughly enjoyed their visit and had time to explore some of the sights of Rome, as well as seeing the first -rate film.

In April 1975 Wendy and I stayed at Benedicta Whistler's flat in Blackheath. The weather was mixed with rain, hail and snow during the week but it didn't stop us visiting the Royal Observatory and Cutty Sark, and the painted hall and chapel at the Royal Naval College in Greenwich. Other visits were to Westminster Abbey and the Tate gallery, and we took a river bus from Greenwich to Westminster pier. I had to pace myself and rest when needed.

We visited Morley's early music shop in Lewisham to see and price their virginals and harpsichords. A friend had lent me a virginals and I found the keys much easier to depress than piano keys, but the cost was well outside my budget. On our way back to Birmingham we visited Fenton House in Hampstead where there was an interesting collection of early musical instruments including virginals, harpsichords, spinets and square pianos; some we could play.

Pembrokeshire was the destination for our summer holiday in June: Wendy and I stayed at the bungalow of Bishop Mark Green's sister at Llangwm near Haverfordwest (Mark was suffragan Bishop of Aston in Birmingham). It was very hot and we enjoyed the refreshing sea breeze near the coast. We explored St David's with its ancient cathedral set in a hollow, then on to Whitesands Bay to paddle and cool ourselves. Fishguard, Strumblehead, Broadhaven and Dale proved interesting seaside towns and Haverfordwest was useful for shopping. On our last day we had an exciting boat trip around Ramsay Island where we saw seals, guillemots and razorbills, and afterwards went to the restaurant at St David's Palace for tea.

※ *Confusion* ※

Barbara and Derek Acock, who had moved to Gloucester invited me to stay with them for the duration of the Three Choirs Festival. Derek, who has a fine counter tenor voice, was singing with the Cathedral choir, being a lay clerk. We were treated to a performance of *The Dream of Gerontius* and Bernstein's *Chichester Psalms*, as well as the regular office services of Matins and Evensong, and a sung Eucharist. I met several of their friends, also Sheila Patterson, a former colleague at the physiotherapy department at Birmingham General Hospital.

Wendy and I returned to Benedicta's flat in Blackheath for a few days in the autumn. This time we visited Kenwood House in Hampstead and saw the magnificent paintings by Gainsborough, and the Victoria and Albert Museum where we saw several Constable paintings and parts of their costume and musical instrument collections. We also went to a concert at the Queen Elizabeth Hall. At Greenwich we returned to the National Maritime museum, and took the boat from Greenwich to Westminster pier and thence to the National Gallery. On our last day I took Wendy to Southwark Cathedral, reminding me of my childhood links. She was very interested to see the memorial to William Shakespeare, having been an actress when young.

Later in the year Wendy drove us to Liverpool where we stayed with Doris and Hazel Kabity. I visited Dorothy Stewart who was very frail but in good spirits. We walked on Otterspool promenade by the river Mersey and saw improvements which had been made since we lived there. The next day we had a short walk at Formby beach, windy as always, to show Wendy some of our favourite places when we lived in Great Crosby.

In Spring 1976 I briefly visited Gladys Pichler at Orpington so I could attend a concert at the Fairfield Halls in Croydon, where Frank Wibaut was giving a recital. He played brilliantly and was pleased to see me in the audience with Mrs Jacqueline Jefferies, one of our tutors at King's with whom I had kept in touch. Gladys took me out for a meal at Dickens and Jones after shopping there, a revelation as I wasn't used to extravagant living.

※ *Walking on Wheels* ※

A month later I went with my parents to a small village called Knill, near Kington on the border of Shropshire and Wales to stay with Margaret Shotton, an obstretician and gynaecologist, who worked in Birmingham and had met Father. A part of the country previously unknown to me, the well-wooded hills were spectacular with spring flowers. We walked, enjoyed pub lunches, and relaxed. We were introduced to the local vicar, Stanley Trickett, and his wife who had invited Father to preach for the morning service at the ancient church of Old Radnor, part of the Knill parish. We went to Hereford Cathedral for evensong and were impressed by the choir's singing. Stanley Trickett's daughter had her own pony and I was encouraged to have a ride, which was fun and a new experience. Some years later I was surprised to meet Stanley Trickett in Salisbury; he had moved to be vicar of Shrewton parish church in Wiltshire, and later he and his wife retired to Salisbury.

12
Problem Solved ~ Diagnosis July – December 1976

Introduction

ON SUNDAY 18TH July 1976 I travelled from Birmingham by coach to London where Mrs Gordon Davies, wife of Canon Davies who had worked with Father at Southwark Cathedral, met me at the coach station. She drove me to King's College Hospital where I was admitted to Trundle ward, the same ward and even the same bed position as when I was a patient in 1962. Professor Anderson had warned me that my stay might be prolonged as he would not let me go home until a diagnosis had been made, and the staff were told to fill my time with useful activities.

I had contacted several London friends before leaving home and Caragh Hanning visited me on the first evening. She suggested bringing a scrabble board with her and we subsequently enjoyed a series of brain teasing games. When I was allowed out at weekends she took me to her Blackheath home for tea, reminding me of earlier times when I babysat for her son James in the 1950s. We walked on the heath and in Greenwich Park where the autumn trees were wonderful shades of yellow and brown.

In hospital I helped the nurses with morning and evening drinks and after a week or so did the rounds on my own, having learnt the different dietary allowances and preferences of the patients. Some had diabetes or were on restricted diets, and others not allowed to drink before an anaesthetic.

I could walk round the hospital and to WH Smith's in the main corridor to purchase newspapers for some of the patients, visited the physiotherapy department to see Mrs Jacqueline Jefferies who was on the teaching staff when I trained at King's, and had coffee with the other members of staff. Jacqueline took me to her home for an evening meal, followed by some weeding in the garden which gave me a taste of normal life and a break from hospital routine.

I found peace and calm in the hospital chapel and when the priest knew I enjoyed playing the piano he invited me to practice. The nurses also let me practice in their sitting room, but the keys of both pianos were rather stiff for my weak fingers. I attended lunchtime concerts in the chapel, the Musical Society concerts in the evening, and midweek evensongs.

I occasionally went shopping at Camberwell Green, sometimes needing to take the bus back if tired. Gluten free bread, which was prescribed a short time after I had been in hospital, I found rather tasteless so bought a toaster, which certainly improved things. Soon I was toasting other patients' bread.

At weekends and in the evenings I walked to nearby Ruskin Park for fresh air and to see the colourful display of flowers. I found it refreshing to have freedom and mental space after the noise of the hospital and its stuffy atmosphere. The weather was exceptionally hot, so I sat on the ward balcony overlooking the main line trains to Victoria, and Ruskin Park beyond. There was some shade but my knees were not protected and got sunburnt, which caused amusement.

I made friends with the staff at the Voluntary Research charity shop and as Christmas approached was asked to help sell cards and gifts to visitors and patients during the rush at midday. All profits from the shop went towards funding hospital medical research.

I went to the occupational therapy department to use an electric typewriter for my own letters as well as typing some of their paperwork;

at weekends the typewriter was brought to the ward. Auntie Margaret brought a clarinet and tutorial book for me to try playing, as it was difficult to blow my bassoon with enough force. A small office near the ward was allocated for these activities after 5pm during the week and at weekends. I was also put to work doing basic woodwork and made a window box and later kettle tippers for safe pouring, one of which I took home to use myself. As my muscles were weak I was given the less strenuous task of finishing off wooden articles and filing rough edges. I became an expert at finishing off raised wooden toilet seats. A static bicycle which operated a wood saw was used to strengthen my legs. I continued with my tapestry, which I had brought with me and after completing several small pictures, patchwork was suggested as an alternative. Eventually I made a sizeable tablecloth using Laura Ashley pieces, which an occupational therapist brought for me. Before I went home she took me shopping to Oxford Street to buy new clothes and gifts for Christmas.

My back problem was treated by a physiotherapist with hydrotherapy in a very warm pool (96° F) and not large enough for swimming, but suitable for specific exercises which were increased in difficulty. I met other patients and particularly a young Canadian child, suffering from Still's disease (childhood rheumatoid arthritis), whom I visited on the children's ward and was invited to her birthday party. As a result I was asked to read to other young children.

Visitors

I MISSED MY FAMILY and friends but visitors were a great help. Father came every week, bringing post and clean clothes. When he stayed in London for meetings he visited more often and both parents came after the Buckingham Palace Garden party looking very glamorous. On another occasion Father brought Sir Arthur Chetwynd and his wife with him having met them in London for a meal. Later my parents visited on their way to Canterbury Cathedral for the installation of a friend as a Canon. Mother sent fresh fruit and foods she knew I liked to supplement my diet. Gladys Pichler from Orpington visited regularly and sometimes Mother stayed with her when she was in London. Petrena and Michael, who sent me light novels, visited when they could and Elisabeth and Brian came regularly from their home in St Albans sometimes with nieces Sarah and Rachel (James was away at boarding school). When I was allowed out at weekends they took me to the Royal Festival Hall and the South Bank. Wendy Beavis wrote regularly and she and the Health visitor, Mrs Clark from Birmingham, also came. So did my cousin, Sue Hampson, who lived in Friern Barnet, north London and Aunt Ruth, when she was in London. Mrs Davies and her husband took me back to their home in central London, and on one occasion we went for a walk by the Serpentine in Hyde Park.

Both Freda Critchley, when she stayed with Auntie at Bishop's Croft, and Tessa Hollis, daughter of Archdeacon Hollis who assisted Father with administration of the diocese, came to see me. Benedicta Whistler introduced me to Biddy Carrick, a friend who taught at a boarding school in Surrey and she became a friend of mine, with whom I spent many holidays at her retirement cottage in Stratton, north Cornwall. Other visitors included Margaret Jenkinson, whose flat I had taken over when a student at King's, Joy Whiting Smith, a physiotherapist at Birmingham General Hospital, Muriel Elphick from the Chartered Society of Physiotherapy Member's Benevolent Fund, with whom I kept in touch until her death, Dr Hearn from Birmingham, Elisabeth's school friend Susan Wilson, who became Susan Williamson and showed me her wedding photographs, and Daisy and Fred from Luton with my godmother, Kathleen Weston.

Former patients returned to see me including an elderly lady Ada Buxton who lived nearby; we later corresponded until her death. A young and lively teenager Nicky with whom I had shared the double side ward, brought her sisters and we played scrabble.

✽ Problem Solved ✽

Maggie Allerton brought her young baby who would sit on our beds and cheer us with his chatter. He is now a father and I hear about his family when Maggie writes at Christmas.

When Father drove to London he took me out to Dulwich Park where we admired the well-kept gardens and massive trees. In August my parents told me they had at last found a suitable house to rent for retirement in Salisbury. Tony Stroud with whom they were staying, suggested a very old, converted chapel which belonged to the Trustees of St Nicholas Hospital of which he was one. It was small and in a poor state of repair but within walking distance of the Cathedral and town, and my parents liked the location on a small island on the river Avon. There were two living rooms and three bedrooms and they decided to take it in preparation for Father's retirement on his 70th birthday, 1st November 1977.

Father had contacted his second cousins, Dorothy (known as Doffy) Allan and her sister Vera Brown who lived in North Harrow

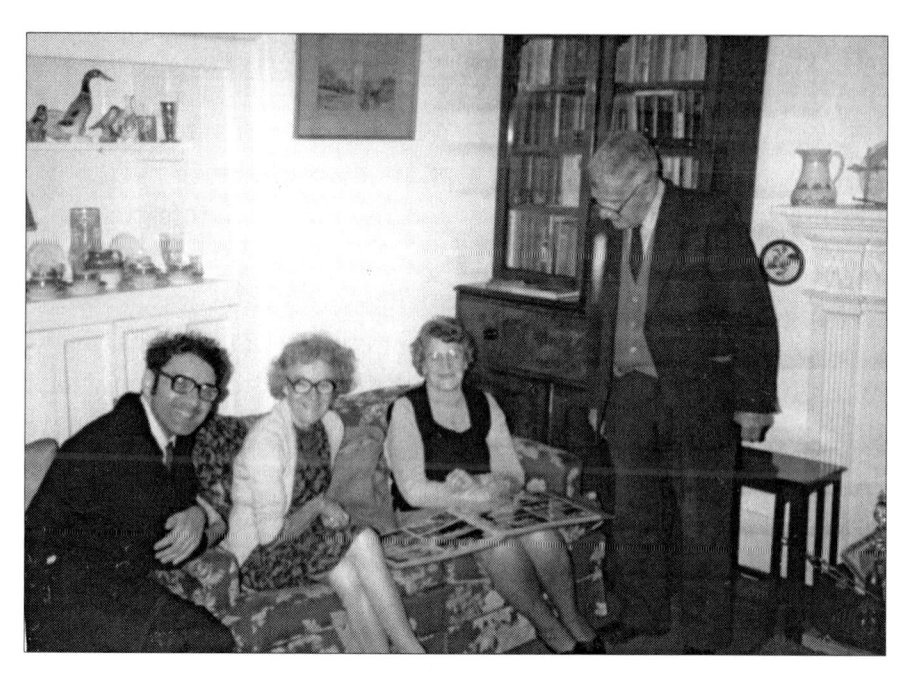

Father with Vera, Doffy and Martin

and Pinner respectively. They often came at weekends usually with the former's son, Martin. We either went to Brockwell Park in Herne Hill or Dulwich, or by bus into central London. We looked at the masterpieces in Dulwich art gallery, and the interesting musical instruments and masks as well as other treasures in the Horniman museum. On a trip to Lewisham we went to Morleys for me to try playing a clavichord because the keys were much lighter to touch than a piano, but I was disappointed by the tone. We went to St Paul's Cathedral which I hadn't visited since moving north, and Westminster Cathedral; we walked on the South Bank and had tea at the Festival Hall, and I took them to Southwark Cathedral and London Bridge and showed them the Borough Market. After Martin was confirmed we shared a Holy Communion service in the hospital Chapel. I looked forward to the weekend outings, which were a good break from hospital routine and kept me in touch with the reality of the outside world.

Personal Health

As the weeks went by with no positive results from the tests I became despondent, but kept up my morale with purposeful activities at occupational therapy and the voluntary research shop, and frequent visitors.

Despite the uncertainty of moving to different wards several times during my stay, occupational therapy and physiotherapy gave me some stability and security. Eventually I was moved to a new block and had a single room in William Bowman ward. Most patients were in hospital for treatments to their eyes, but there were several 'lodgers' from other departments. My small room was well equipped with en suite facilities, a wardrobe and a wide window ledge for books. I dressed every day and felt more relaxed and as though I was in a hotel. The staff allowed me into the ward kitchen to make hot drinks for visitors, which was a special privilege for patients.

✽ Problem Solved ✽

I was seen by Professor Robert Cawley, a distinguished psychiatrist from the Maudesley hospital, who after several consultations declared that I had no signs of a psychosomatic disease and that my illness was definitely physical, which reassured me about my mental state. But after the stress of the past few months I had become depressed and was prescribed chlorpromazine (Largactil), as well as anabolic steroids to build up my muscles. A week later both drugs were discontinued because of untoward side effects; I felt sick and very spaced out again. I was put on a high protein and gluten free diet to try and alleviate my digestive problems which were thought to be due to certain food intolerances. Two weeks later I tried eating ordinary bread again but that caused more diarrhoea so had to go back to gluten free bread.

The next useful event was a thorough neurological examination by Professor David Parkes, who asked for electromyographs, which revealed a neurophysiological defect in the muscles. At last there were clues to my illness. Then a muscle biopsy was taken from my left shoulder under a local anaesthetic. This was extremely painful and I needed extra painkillers for several days and couldn't attend hydrotherapy until the incision healed. The muscle biopsy was normal but the problem was found to be at the neuromuscular junction. The diagnosis was proximal and distal spinal muscular atrophy, an extremely rare condition hence the difficulty in diagnosis which had taken four years. It was similar to progressive poliomyelitis (though not from the polio virus) and only five other patients in the world had been reported. The ultimate prognosis was unknown. My own feelings were mixed: relief that I knew what I had to cope yet with concerns about my future. Little did I know until after Father's death that in a letter Professor Anderson had told my parents that the prognosis was not good and that by the time I was 60 I would probably be totally paralysed. I found the letter when I was 53, and resolved then to prove him wrong.

I was given time to think about the future and came to the conclusion that there were two alternatives: self pity and wallow in gloom about my future, or fight and get on with life as fully as possible despite my limitations. I chose the latter. Although I could never return to work I wouldn't be beaten and dictated to by my disease; I would exercise to keep active and maintain muscle strength as long as possible though resting between activities when needed. Life would be different but I would make the best of what I could do and be positive. I had supportive parents and many good friends, and would take up new interests.

The first was to join the Seecham Group, my local branch of the Riding for the Disabled Association (RDA) which I had recommended to many young patients over the years; if my legs wouldn't allow me to enjoy country walks I could travel by horseback. I had many happy years riding with the RDA and when that became impossible, because of increased back pain, joined Carriage Driving for Disabled, continuing my love of animals and the countryside. There was always time to notice different insects and birds, cobwebs and wild flowers, and to listen to bird song. Over the next years I wrote several articles about the benefits of riding and carriage driving for disabled people which were published in the RDA and Carriage Driving magazines, the *British Medical Journal* and *Physiotherapy*, the journal of the Chartered Society of Physiotherapy and others.

A psychiatrist from Professor Cawley's team visited to see how I had taken news of the diagnosis, and we discussed future plans. The dietician also came as it had been established that my digestive problems were definitely due to food intolerance; she helped me plan my diet when I was allowed home and gave me recipes for which King's would supply the gluten free flour. I would collect a sack at my out-patient appointments, and later arrangements were made for the flour to be delivered by carrier.

Professor Anderson wouldn't allow me home for several weeks after the diagnosis so I carried on my usual activities helping on the ward, working in occupational therapy and doing exercises in hydrotherapy. I bought Christmas cards from the Voluntary Research

Problem Solved

shop, wrote those and attended carol services in the hospital chapel. My parents and I discussed plans for Christmas and New Year, only three weeks away.

On December 11th Professor Anderson told me I could go home the following week. He prescribed a capsule, cromoglycate (Intal), which was placed in the centre of a spin inhaler where its coating was pierced. I then took a deep breath in, which caused the tiny fan inside to release the powder into my lungs. This was used to treat auto-immune diseases which were thought to be part of my problem.

I returned home on December 18th, five months after my admission to King's, the problem solved, and looking forward to the future. Life would certainly be different but I was determined to be positive, keep active and be useful to others despite my physical problems, and what wonderful, happy, exciting and fulfilling years followed.

Epilogue
The Way Forward

THAT WAS IT, I had made my decision and wouldn't be beaten by my illness.

Life goes on: I was still the same person and would carry on doing all I could to live a full life and help others, albeit in a different way from that I had followed as a physiotherapist.

We moved to Salisbury on 1st November 1977, my Father's 70th birthday. Some structural work had already been done to the house before our move but more decoration was needed and our first few weeks were once again spent with the company of builders.

The house, formerly called St John's Chapel on the Isle is a Grade 2 listed building. It was built in the early 13th Century to provide accommodation and food to pilgrims who had crossed the ford through the river Avon, which runs by the Chapel, on their route between Winchester and Wilton, the two major towns on the pilgrimage route. In 1245, Bishop Bingham, of Salisbury, built a bridge over the Avon by the Chapel. He and the Clergy of Old Sarum had by then decided to build their new Cathedral on low ground near the river, and the city of New Sarum was becoming established around their new Cathedral. St Nicholas Hospital, founded in 1215, an ancient order for pilgrims, had been established next to the Chapel, so those needing assistance were given food and a bed there, taking over the function of the Chapel. The next mention of the Chapel in record books is early in 1500, and again in the nineteenth century when it was used as a library for Canon Christopher Wordsworth, then Master of St Nicholas Hospital. The

Epilogue

Chapel, with its 3-foot walls on the garden and ground floor levels, was converted into a house and the Spire removed in the nineteenth century, and a first floor with normal thickness walls was added at that time. Two of the three original Early English lancet windows remain on the east wall, with the third one being filled in, together with several others around the house, probably at the time of the window tax in the 18th century. A double Piscina (washing basin and a relic of the former Chapel) remains at the east end of the basement. Despite the alterations the former Chapel retains its character, with a small secluded garden on the east side. The original ground floor, on river level, isn't suitable for habitation but ideal for storage and garden equipment, and although we had disposed of many items of furniture before leaving Birmingham, we stored the surplus, together with garden equipment and my wheelchairs there. It took us time to adjust to living in the house with its small kitchen, living and dining rooms on the ground floor with three bedrooms, a bathroom and toilets on the first floor, after the spaciousness of Bishop's Croft, but we knew we had made the right move.

By New Year we felt more settled and ready to start our new lives. Father was approached by the Bishop of Salisbury, George Reindorp, with whom he had worked in the Southwark Diocese, to be Priest-in Charge of three small villages, Odstock, Nunton and Bodenham about two miles from Salisbury. The position was for six months. Father accepted, glad to get back to the roots of his ministry as a parish priest, and was so happy he stayed for seven years. Mother was pleased to be settled and have a

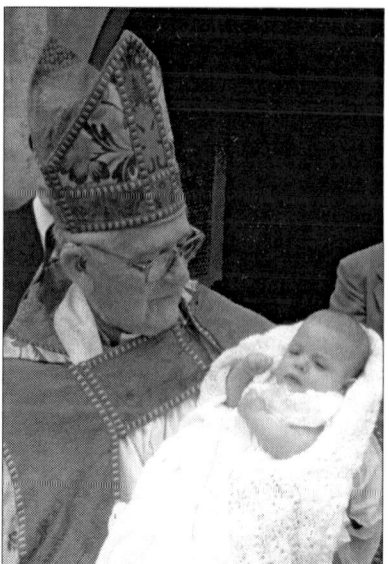

Father having Christened a baby at Nunton Church

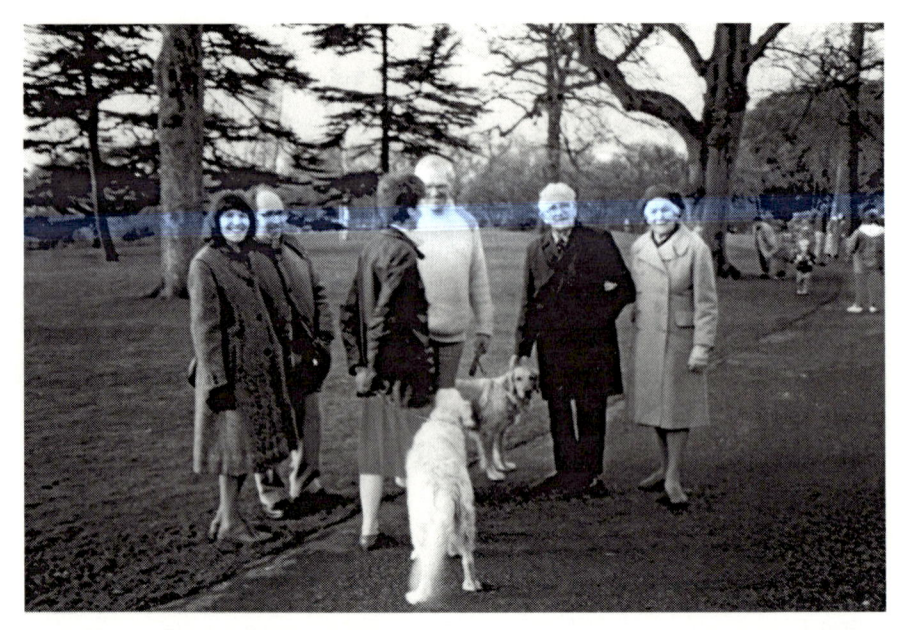

My sisters and husbands out walking with my parents on a visit to Salisbury. Left to right: Petrena with Michael, Elisabeth and Brian with their dogs and my parents.

small house and garden to take care of.

My parents were wonderful, caring for my sisters and me throughout our childhood, and when I became ill they continued supporting and encouraging me to do all I could.

Before leaving Birmingham I had been introduced to Wilton House Riding for the Disabled and within a couple of weeks of our move I was driven by a Wilton volunteer back to the National Agricultural Centre at Stoneleigh in the Midlands. I had been invited to speak at the Annual conference of the Riding for the Disabled Association about my experience of changing from a working physiotherapist to a rider with Riding for Disabled.

I continued weekly riding sessions at Wilton. In summer we rode round the spacious grounds of Wilton House, the home of the Pembroke family. When it was wet we rode in the original stables belonging to the house. Pat Burgess, our leader and instructor was, and still is, an inspiration to all who meet her and everyone enjoyed and

✳ Epilogue ✳

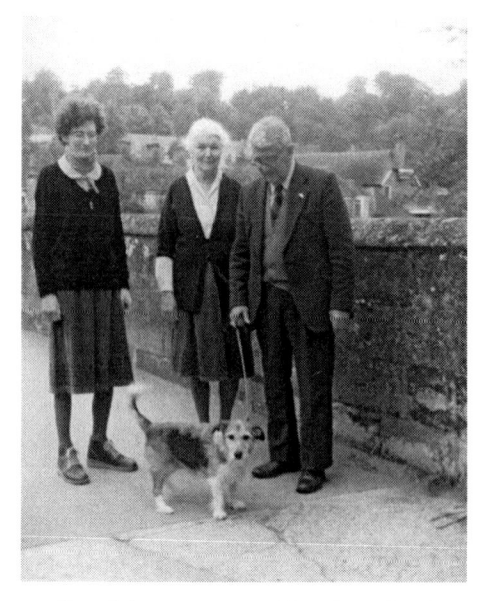

Jill with her parents on Harnham bridge

benefited greatly from sessions. Volunteers were encouraging and after some months one helper, Louise Fry, whose horse I rode, invited me to her stables at nearby Stratford Tony. I rode around the lanes and bridle paths, which saved her taking her pony to Wilton each week, and gave me a variety of rides in the beautiful countryside. I loved it and continued riding until the jolting hurt my back intolerably.

In 1988, a neighbour, the late Morna MacLaren, mentioned she had heard of a new group of Carriage Driving for Disabled at nearby Longford Park, in Bodenham. She had been in the Land Army and an enthusiastic rider and offered to be my helper and drive me to Bodenham. By this time I was unable to drive a car because of lack of strength in my neck and arms. At the stables we helped harness the pony, then my wheelchair would be loaded into the cart via a ramp at the rear and off we would go around the lanes of Lord Radnor's estate, enjoying the scenes and scents of the countryside. We had a great team of helpers and drivers. Each turnout (pony and cart) had double reins, one set for the disabled driver and one for an accompanying driver who took as much, or as little, control of the pony and cart as was needed. Two outriders, usually on bicycles, one in front and the other behind each cart, went with each turnout for safety purposes. Morna and I thoroughly enjoyed each session, seeing the countryside at various times of the year and in all weathers.

The stables at Longford Castle were old and full of fascination, and on wet days we cleaned harness, familiarising ourselves with the

Walking on Wheels

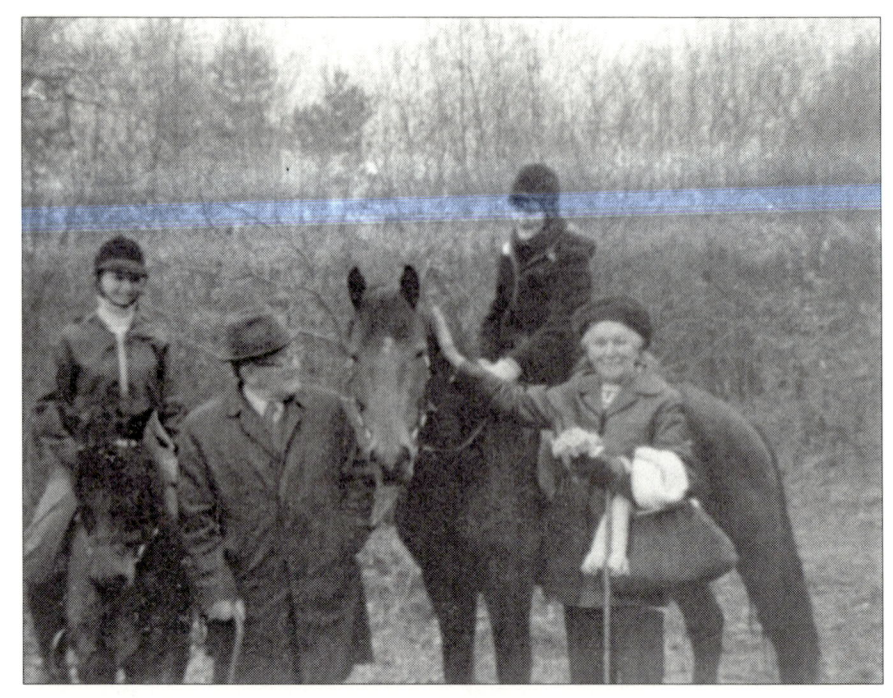

Jill on horseback

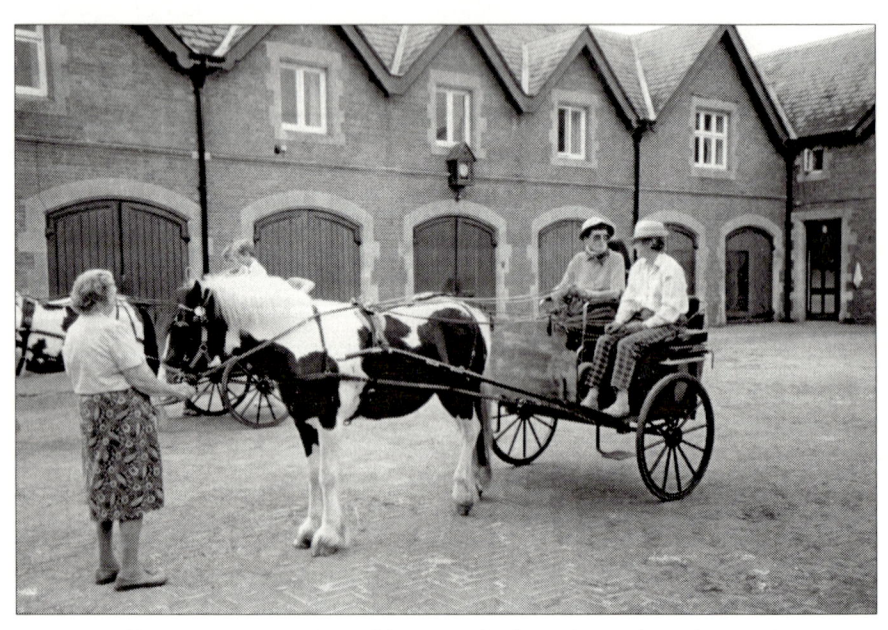

Jill in a carriage at the stables, Longford Castle, ready to drive off.

* Epilogue *

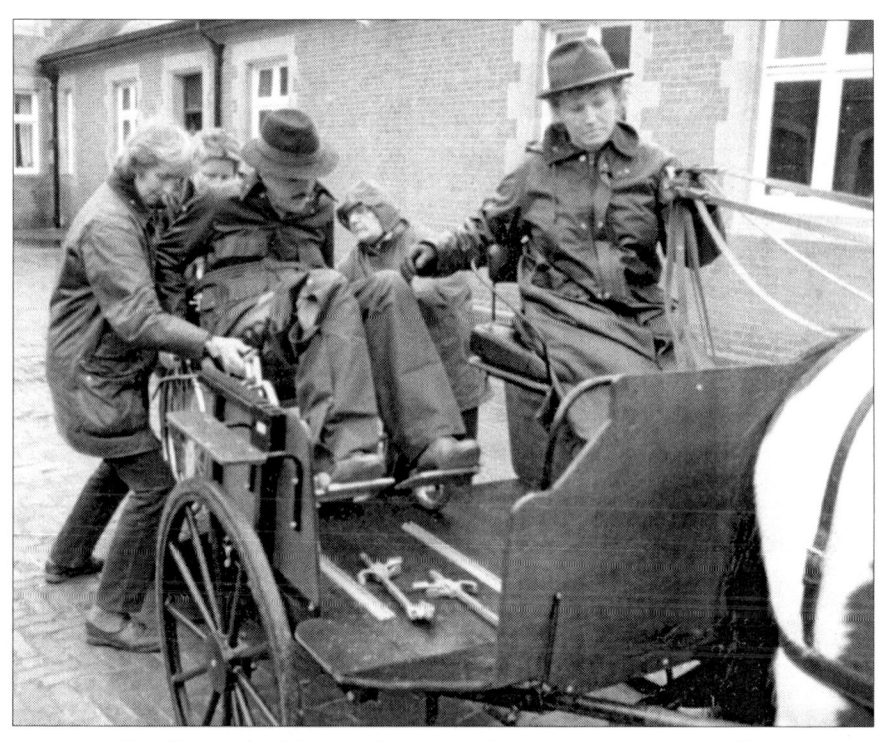

Loading a wheelchair and occupant into a carriage at the stables

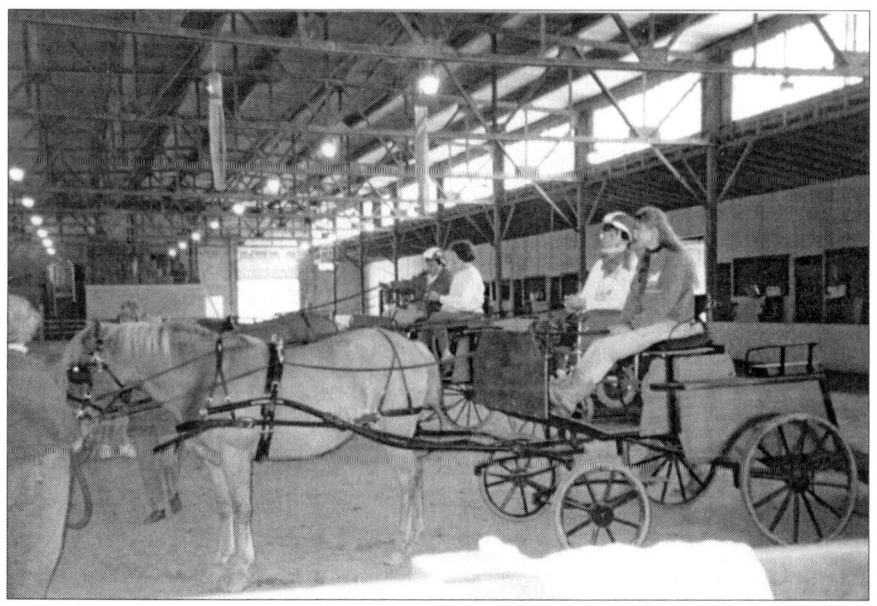

Jill ready to drive off in the indoor driving arena, Maryland, USA

names of the various parts of the equipment and so learning to tack up a pony. Apart from the practical advantage, it was all necessary knowledge for passing the Preliminary exam of the British Driving Society for Disabled Drivers, which I achieved in 1991.

Our group entered drivers for the Riding for Disabled Association (RDA), and the British Driving Society (BDS) annual shows, held in Windsor Great Park. The days out were great fun whether competing or going as a spectator and one year we were presented to HRH the Princess Royal, who is Patron of the Riding for the Disabled Association. At the British Driving Society Show we enjoyed watching other drivers, some driving Shetlands, others with tandems (one pony following and harnessed with a leader) or randems (three ponies), and between times watched polo matches taking place nearby. I have a good collection of rosettes from both the RDA and BDS events. We also met together at Longford Castle or other suitable venues, for Christmas lunch.

After a few years the group had to move to West Grimstead stables, a few miles east of Salisbury, where we drove in lanes and parkland belonging to the farm. Spring drives were memorable for a route through wonderful bluebell woods; the scent and colour were unforgettable. By this time Morna was unable to help but another friend, John Roe, stepped in as my helper.

I was interested in carriage driving around the world and did research into this, making contacts in several countries. This led to an invitation to visit USA and the Maryland group of Carriage Driving. In April 1994, after months of work and fund raising, a very good friend, Jenny Barrett and I set off to Washington DC where we stayed with Vivian, a fellow member of Travelling Talk, a group of disabled people around the world who welcomed disabled people to their country. Richard Branson generously sponsored the project, giving us free upper class flights to Boston, and the Chartered Society of Physiotherapy awarded me a grant to help with other costs. We flew from Boston to Washington DC where we stayed for twelve days

※ Epilogue ※

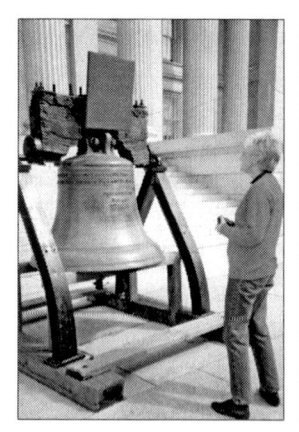

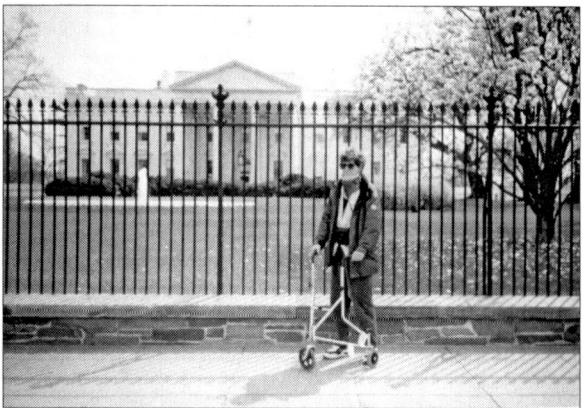

(left) Jenny Barrett by the Independence Bell, Washington; (right) Jill outside The White House, Washington, DC, USA

in a suburb of the city with Vivian, exploring that interesting city and spending a day with the Maryland group of Carriage Driving for Disabled, observing the similarities and differences between our groups. We travelled by local buses and Metro which were far advanced compared to the transport in UK for wheelchair users at that time and visited the White House, Capitol, Cathedral, Mall and several of the wonderful museums and art galleries. Vivian, our hostess, took us on an evening dinner cruise up the Potomac river which borders one side of Washington DC with interesting views of the City.

On my return I wrote papers for our sponsors and for Riding for the Disabled Association who were most interested in the venture. I wrote articles for several of the Carriage Driving magazines also *Physiotherapy, Therapy Weekly* and *Travelling Talk.*

The Longford Park group continued until 1996 when sadly it was forced to close because of lack of volunteers. By then I was unable to take much control of the turnout because of increasing weakness in my arms. I have very happy memories of my years of riding and carriage driving and several articles about the therapeutic benefits of riding and carriage driving were published in both riding and carriage driving magazines, the Association of Disabled Professionals Bulletin, and medical journals including *Therapy Weekly, Physiotherapy* and the Christmas 1990 issue of the *British Medical Journal*.

I could continue swimming and met many new friends at the pool at Salisbury District Hospital, which I joined soon after our move. Thirty years later I still swim there regularly. Although I have to use floats and other aids now and my stroke is not like any other, it doesn't matter: I am keeping my joints supple and muscles as strong as the disease allows. Over the years I have done several sponsored swims: for Muscular Dystrophy, Salisbury Cathedral Spire Appeal, and latterly for charities supported by the Salisbury Rotary Club annual Swimathon. In 2005, Dogs for the Disabled benefited from the event and Yates, my Dog for the Disabled, and I were presented with a cheque for £2,500 for the charity. I will continue taking part as long as I am able to.

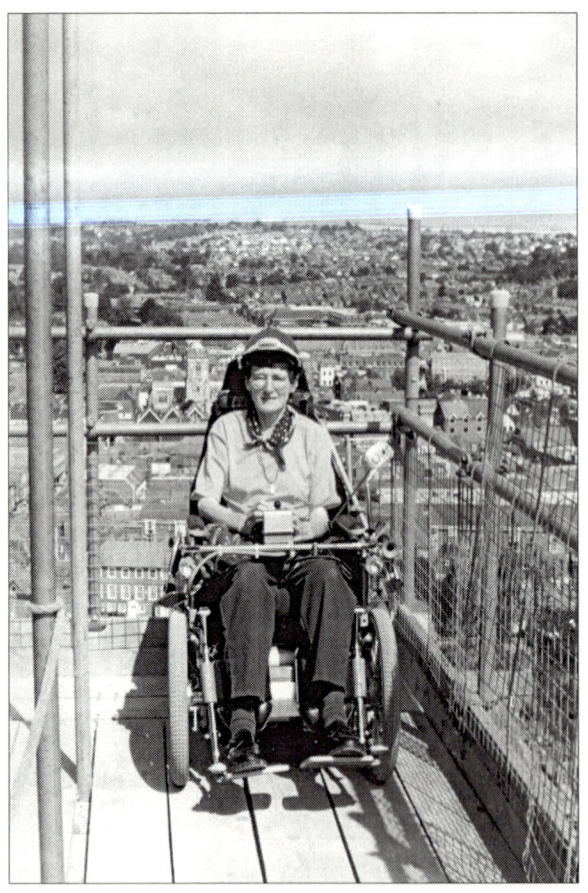

Jill in the work's department lift at the time of the restoration of the Spire of Salisbury Cathedral, looking out over the Cathedral and Salisbury

In 1978 I read that REMAP (Rehabilitation Engineer Movement Advisory Panel) were looking for volunteers. REMAP organisations are nationwide and volunteers work to make or adjust any equipment for elderly and disabled people which cannot be bought 'off the shelf'. I volunteered my previous experience of working as a physiotherapist and an interest in gadgets which could help patients,

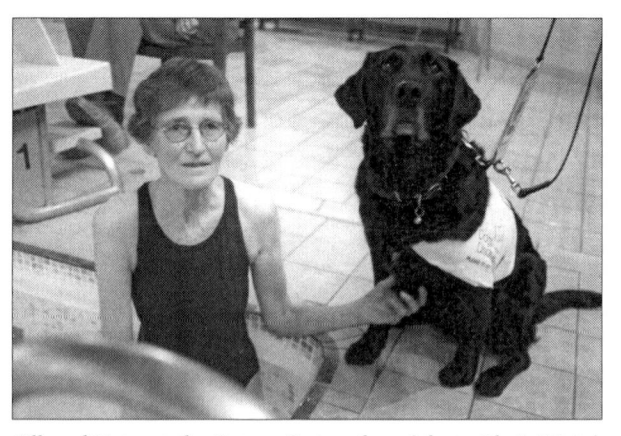

Jill and Yates at the Rotary Swimathon (photo Chris Wain)

as well as my secretarial skills and was taken aback to be asked to start a group in Salisbury. With help from the regional adviser for REMAP our group is now well established and serving a need, having done over 800 jobs, varying from altering the height of a chair to designing and making a hydraulic hoist for our Salisbury swimming pool. I have benefited myself and daily use several pieces of equipment made by the group, and I trust that my advisory contribution to the quarterly panel meetings is still valued. During the early years I was responsible for publicity and spoke on BBC Radio 4 programme *Does he take Sugar* about our work, my first experience of the media. More recently, I have been appointed treasurer of our group.

Committee Work

IN 1978/79 I was asked by an occupational therapist from Salisbury District Council to help establish a group to improve access to shops, offices, churches and other buildings for people with varying disabilities. There were numerous hazards: a lack of dropped kerbs, steps and heavy doors into public buildings, a lack of accessible telephone boxes (mobile phones were not normal equipment for most people in those days), and little accessible public transport. After much work, contacting the various organisations for people with different disabilities, a committee was formed of an administrator and an architect from the District Council, and volunteers from groups for the blind, deaf, mentally handicapped and physically disabled. Our priority was to make officials aware of the need to provide services accessible to all, as well as funding so that we could make alterations, such as dropped kerbs and ramps to enable those in wheelchairs to get on and off pavements at safe places. At first progress was slow but we drew up maps where we considered alterations a priority, and persuaded the Council to include the work in road repairs and make sure it was carried out.

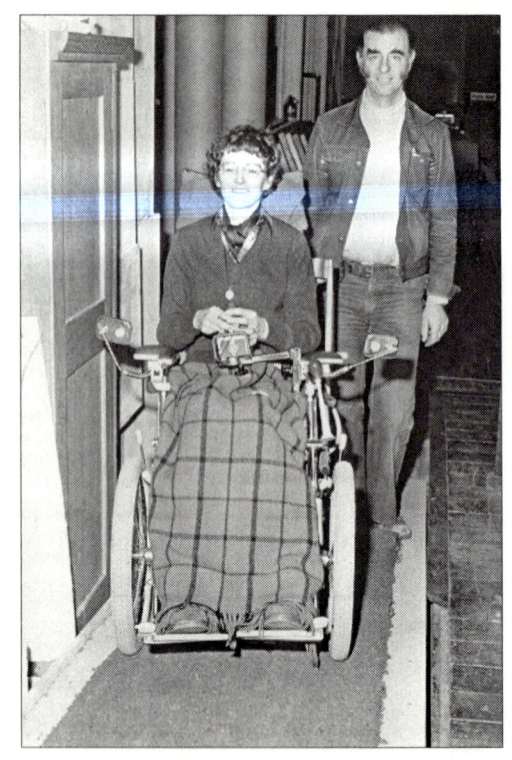

Jill at St Edmund's Art Centre demonstrating easier access to the building as a result of the work done during the International Year of Disabled People.

1981 was designated the International Year of Disabled People and the Mayor at the time, Derek Alford, set up a committee to improve access for disabled people. I was asked to join that committee and we decided to raise funds to make some improvements ourselves. The Cubs did a sponsored walk and raised a good sum of money; I welcomed the boys at the end of their walk. We also asked businesses to do all they could to improve their access.

The main Post Office was a challenge as there were numerous underground cables but eventually work was done and it is now wheelchair friendly.

Epilogue

Other disabilities needed their own alterations, such as devices to assist deaf people and help for those who were blind, and we tried to help.

We encouraged the local bus company and British Rail to make improvements, but we realised changes would take years. At least we had raised awareness of the needs so that work would continue after the official year. Living in an historic city with many listed buildings, some problems have to be tolerated but now in 2011 I can report the situation is vastly improved from that in 1981. With the passing of various stages of the Disability Discrimination Act responsibility has passed to every company, property owner and organisation, but our committee of 1978 certainly helped to initiate improvements.

Following from my volunteer work at the Cheshire home in Herne Hill when I was a student at Kings, 1 visited a Cheshire home near Petersfield, Hampshire, and met several residents. We became friendly and corresponded about our interests and work. In 1980 one of my contacts who was involved in making a film to raise awareness of disability asked if I would take part. This was my first experience of the film and television industry. I was to be filmed showing my friend from the Cheshire home around Salisbury city centre, discussing access to public buildings and facilities. I was invited to the London premiere of the film when I was presented along with the other participants to Lord Snowdon, the President of International Year of Disabled People. The film was shown locally and eventually appeared on national television. Our Access for Disabled committee used it to raise awareness of the needs locally and through it a good sum of money was raised to continue our work.

I had joined the local committee of the Muscular Dystrophy Group in Birmingham after my diagnosis was established, and transferred to the Salisbury branch when we moved. Some members had relatives with the disease and others knew people who had it. We worked hard raising money for research by having 'flag days' around the City centre, sales of donated and second hand goods, and a handball tournament for a few years. This raised considerable sums of money as well as awareness of the condition and I learnt that charity fund raising could be fun as well as hard work. However after several years the committee aged and there wasn't enough support for the group so we had to close.

Interest in music has never waned and I sang with the St John's Singers in Salisbury, for a few years until my lungs weakened and choral singing was impossible. However I was determined to play a wind instrument so bought a clarinet and for a few years had lessons with Libby Poppleton and then Sue De Garis and I enjoyed playing duets with my teacher. As my respiratory muscles weakened, Sue De Garis suggested I play a recorder which requires less force. This has been most successful and has given me great pleasure although I am only able to play for short periods when I have sufficient energy. As well as practising alone I regularly play duets with a friend, Tricia Dragnonetti and at Christmas we join others and go busking in the city centre raising funds for Dogs for the Disabled. I enjoy classical music and am a volunteer programme seller with my dog Yates for concerts given by the Salisbury Musical Society, Salisbury Symphony Orchestra and Salisbury Festival each year.

Thoughout the years I have continued writing papers and many have been published about a variety of topics, including the therapeutic value of music and of yoga, which I did for several years with my very good friend Jenny Barrett. I wrote publicity articles for Salisbury REMAP and several on disability related matters such as the choice of electric wheelchairs. I also reviewed some books for the *British Medical Journal*.

Family Life

My parents were always so supportive that it was a great sadness to realise that my Mother had signs of Alzheimer's

✳ Epilogue ✳

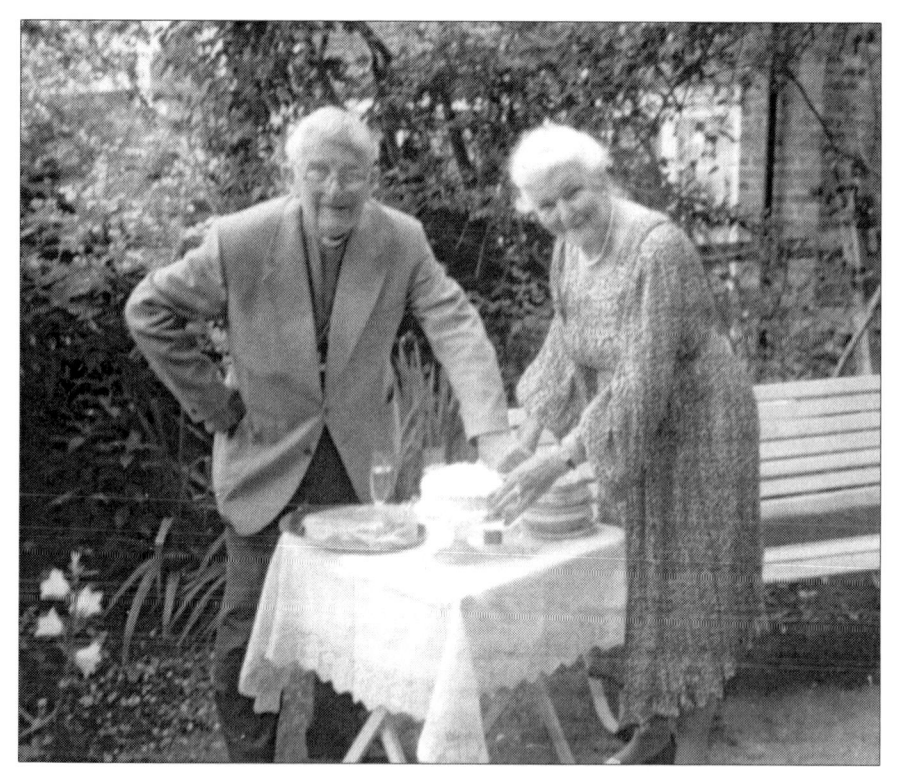

My parents celebrating their golden wedding in happier times.

Disease during the late 1980s. Father and I did our best to manage at home with support from a Community Nurse, but as her condition deteriorated it became harder and after assessment she went to live at a nursing home in Salisbury. By then I was unable to drive but friends took Father and me regularly to visit her; she remained welcoming and loving until her death in 1999. Sadly we realised that Father also had early signs of the disease so he joined Mother, whom he loved so much. Unfortunately he was also diagnosed with a form of epilepsy which complicated other possible treatment and he died in 1994. I was devastated but with support from my friends managed to hide my grief until a year later when my eldest sister, Elisabeth, who had been suffering from a very aggressive form of multiple sclerosis, also died aged 59 years.

Walking on Wheels

My muscles had weakened considerably by then and I needed a lot of help. I couldn't contain my feelings any longer and became very tearful. My GP was most sympathetic and arranged counselling, which helped.

However the biggest factor aiding my recovery was the arrival of my wonderful assistance dog, Astrid. In 1994 I heard about a relatively new charity, Dogs for the Disabled, to which I applied and was accepted and in March 1995 I was partnered with Astrid. The twenty months of waiting seemed very long, but knowledge that I would have my own trained dog cheered me and improved my morale and confidence. I had heard that assistance dogs are trained to help disabled people by retrieving items, pulling and pushing controls and levers, obedience and speaking (barking) on command. All these tasks can be adapted to daily living situations and my dogs have helped me with many tasks using the skills from their training.

When Astrid arrived I was overjoyed. She was very timid at first but so loyal and a wonderful helper. She assisted me with dressing and undressing, pulling shirts, sweaters and socks off, as well as helping me get my arms into jackets and cardigans. She fetched the post and anything I dropped, which relieved my back pain. She opened doors and gates using a rope attached to the handles as well as many other tasks. Her companionship and affection were indescribable and my happiness and confidence soared.

As the years go by, my muscles have deteriorated and my dogs do more and more as the need arises. They ensure I get out for two walks a day (I use my electric wheelchair); it is much more fun taking a dog for a walk than going alone and I have made so many friends because of my dog. People stop and chat, asking about the dog rather than ignoring a person in a wheelchair, and the focus changes from wheelchair to dog. We are asked to give talks to many different groups of people: Brownies, Cubs and Guides, school children of varying ages, Rotary clubs, the Women's Institute and other groups. I have been so thankful to have the benefit of my assistance dog from Dogs

✳ *Epilogue* ✳

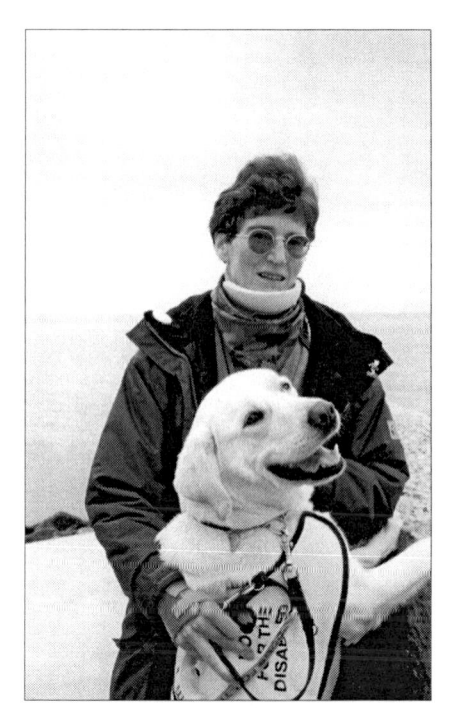

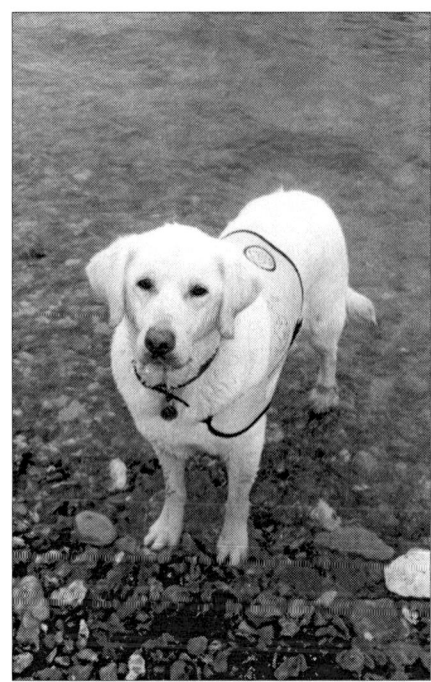

Astrid

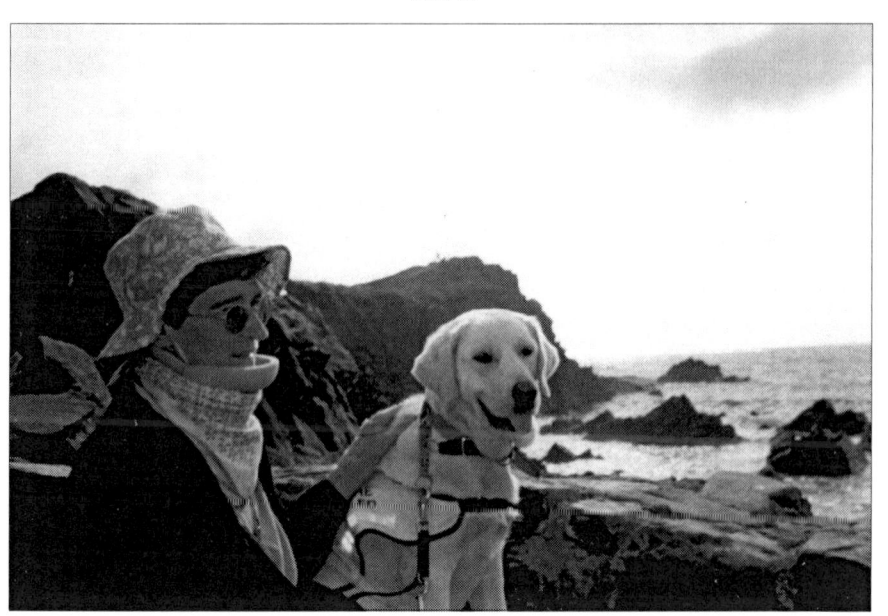

Jill with Astrid on holiday at Hartland Quay, Cornwall

* *Walking on Wheels* *

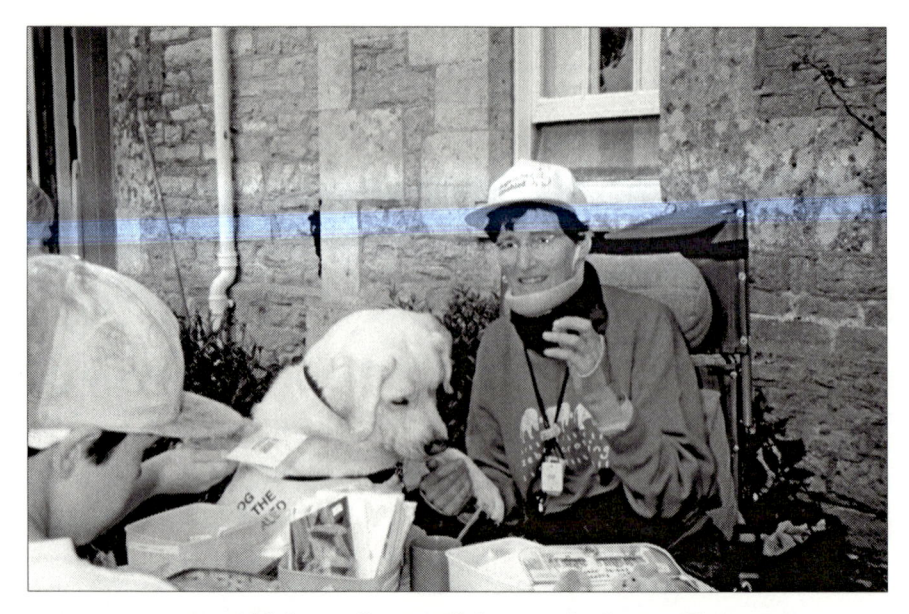

Astrid helping Jill at a stall for Dogs for the Disabled

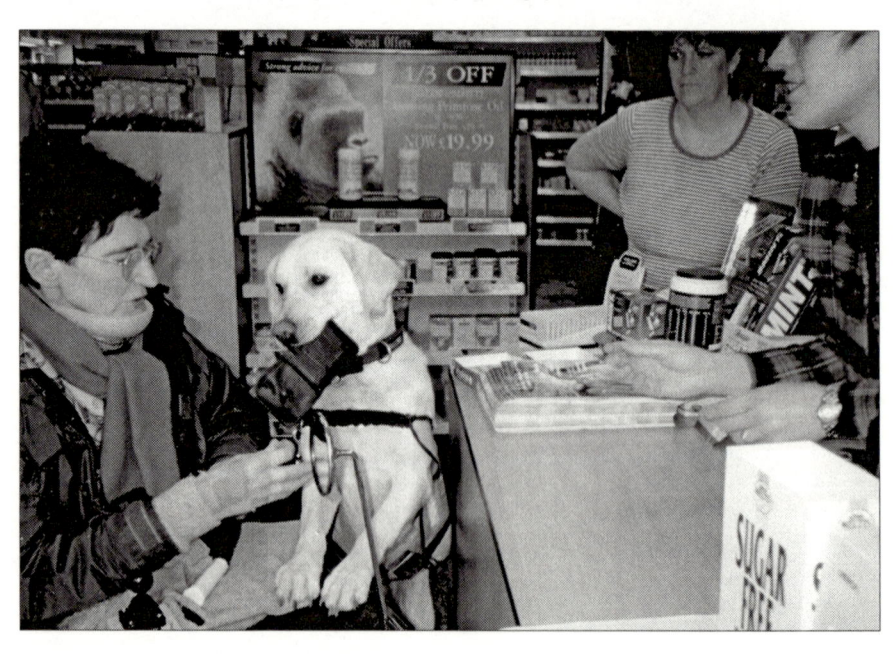

Astrid passing over Jill's purse to the shopkeeper to pay for goods

* Epilogue *

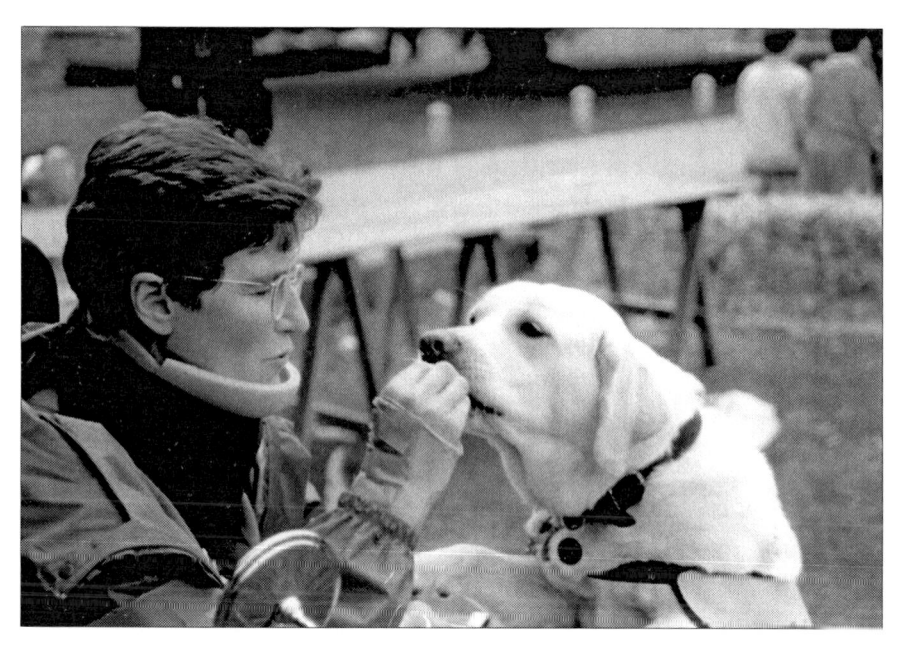

Jill giving Astrid a biscuit reward for helping her.

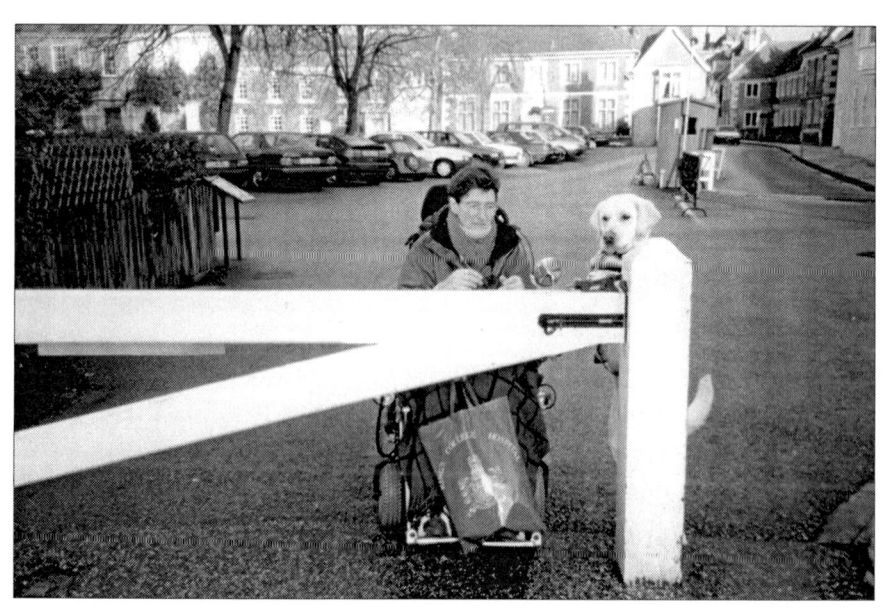

Astrid opening the latch gate in Salisbury Cathdral Close for Jill

for the Disabled that I am glad to give talks and have stalls at fêtes and other events to raise money and awareness of our charity. We meet and come into contact with others with trained dogs, and the world has enlarged so much. Astrid and I were interviewed and televised on two occasions when I was a patient in Southampton General Hospital, and appeared with the TV star Annette Crosbie on a television appeal in aid of our charity, when an amazing sum of money was collected, over £35,000. I was devastated when Astrid became ill with Addison's disease in 2002, but fortunately she pulled through and enjoyed a further fifteen months before a complication of haemolytic anaemia caused her death. My friends were very sad because she had made such an impression on them and they knew how much she meant to me. Without her I felt 'incomplete', whereas with her I felt a 'whole person'.

I didn't dream another dog would mean so much to me until I met Yates, Astrid's successor: he has been a real treasure and a worthy successor. As my health and muscle strength have deteriorated over the years (I am now unable to lift my arms at all nor walk far, and get exhausted very quickly) Yates initially had a long list of tasks that I needed help with, but he is very bright and soon learnt to do all I needed. Even now he learns new and helpful tasks with amazing speed and he is very affectionate. He and I have been interviewed and televised promoting a classical music concert in Salisbury in aid of the charity, and other media interviews.

As the years go by I need more equipment and have been most fortunate in receiving help from charities towards the funding of mobile arm supports and stair lifts. REMAP are always there to make anything which cannot be bought and the rack, which holds my walking aid on the back of my electric wheelchair, is much admired and is an example of the group's work.

Ever since we moved to Salisbury in 1977 I have been a member of the congregation at Salisbury Cathedral. It is a most beautiful, interesting and inspiring building, visited by thousands of people

※ *Epilogue* ※

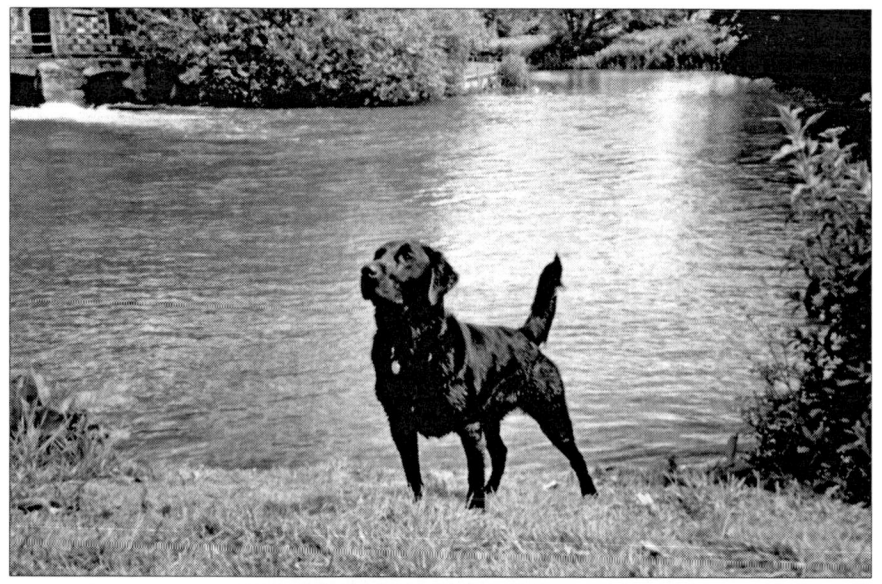

Yates

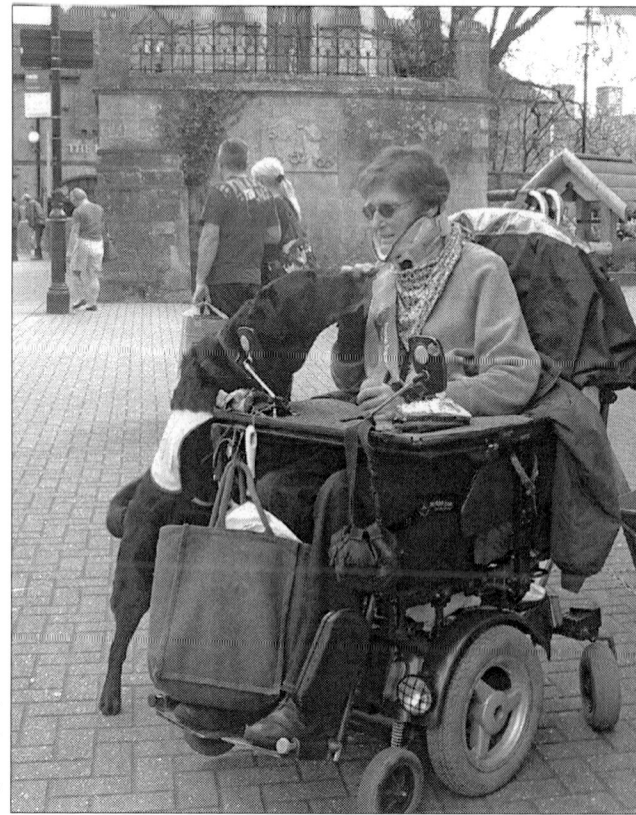

*Yates
receiving praise
having retrieved a
pen I had dropped*

✵ *Walking on Wheels* ✵

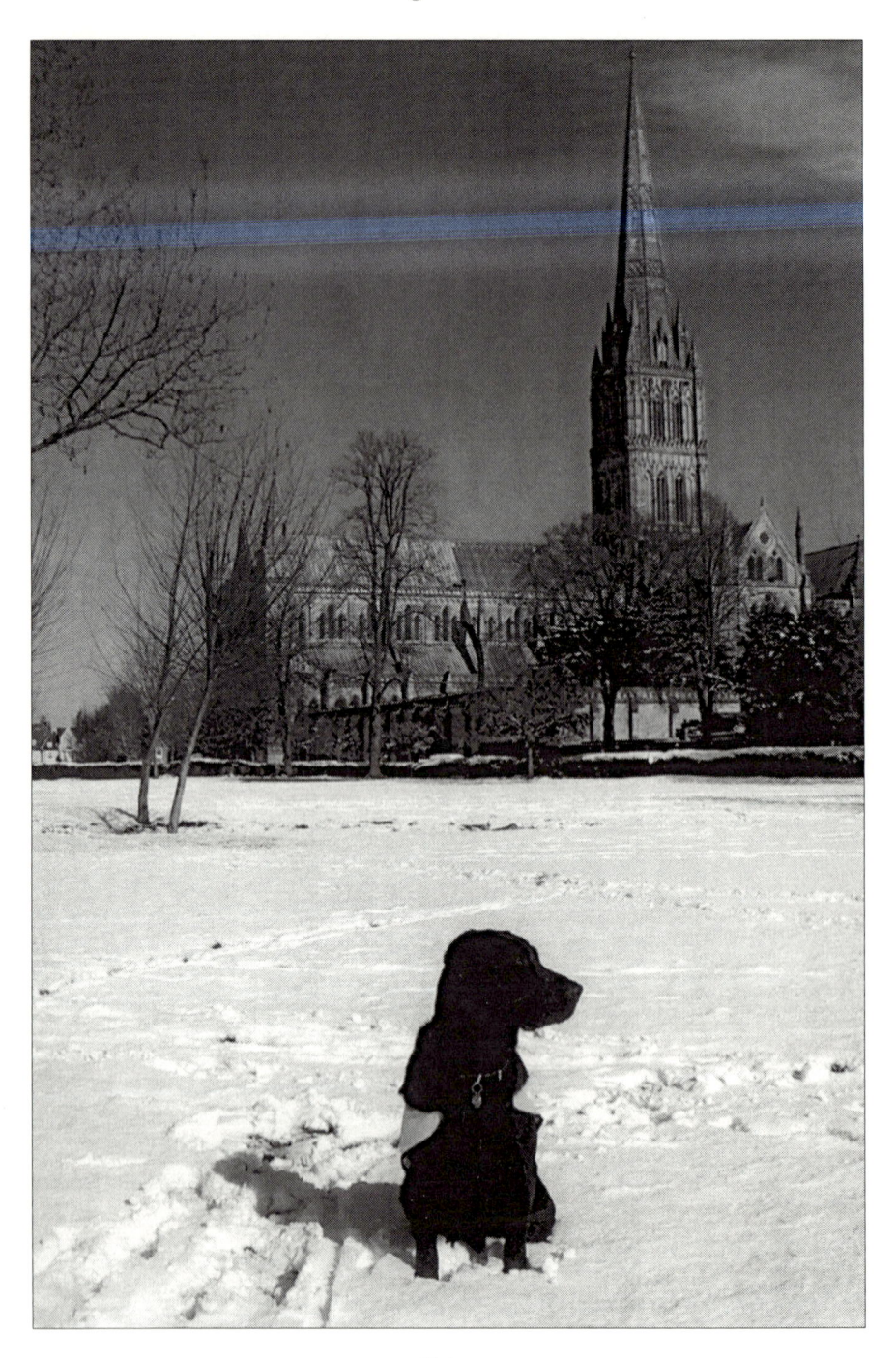

Yates

Epilogue

from around the world every year. I am most fortunate to live within five minutes walk. The music is excellent and over the years we are fortunate to have had talented Directors of Music. The choristers, both boys and girls, are very fond of my dogs and we are invited to go at playtime when the children stroke and relax with my dogs and ask how they help. We also give formal talks when invited by staff, which are enjoyed both by the children and us. Yates and I now help at Sunday school.

I have made many friends through the Cathedral and some now offer to drive us to appointments, or to go to the coast or places of mutual interest. The coast is just an hour's drive from Salisbury and Hengistbury Head is a favourite, along with Mudeford and Highcliffe; further afield we enjoy Tyneham and Studland in Dorset. There are several National Trust properties within easy reach of Salisbury and we enjoy the gardens as well as the architecture and treasures in the stately homes. A talk about churches under the care of the Churches Conservation Trust at U3A led us to visit many in this area and others when on holiday.

For a few years after we moved to Salisbury my parents and I enjoyed several holidays near Bude, north Cornwall staying at the cottage of our family friend, Biddy Carrick. In time my parents preferred to stay at home, and were happy for me to holiday with friends.

Mrs Jenny Barrett from the Cathedral quickly became one of my very good friends. She and her husband have since moved to Barford St Martin, a small village about six miles from Salisbury, and since her retirement from teaching at the Pre Prep department of the Cathedral School we meet each week to go swimming. Jenny had a lively black labrador and in good weather we took the dogs for a walk in the country or to the beach. With Astrid we had several happy holidays in north Cornwall staying with Biddy Carrick. We miss these holidays now, but have enjoyed others in Somerset, Dorset and Cornwall with our dogs. Margaret Lewis, another very good friend and I have had several holidays in South Cornwall, meeting up with Astrid's puppy socialiser, Daphne and her husband David Lambden. (Puppy Socialisers look after Dogs for the Disabled puppies from about eight weeks old, teaching them social behaviour, basic obedience and some taskwork, such as retrieval. This is in preparation for their specialised training when the puppies return to Dogs for the Disabled headquarters at about one year old.).

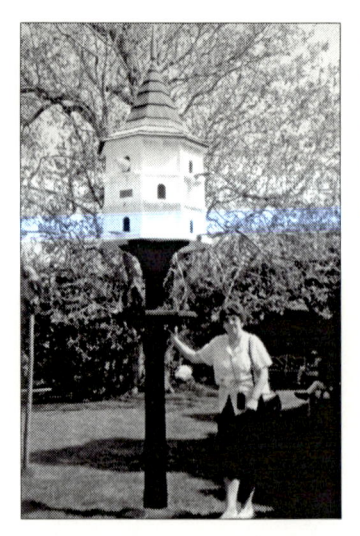

Margaret Lewis at the Lost Gardens of Heligan during one of our holidays in Cornwall

Margaret is a plant expert and we both enjoy going round some of the magnificent gardens, as well as the scenic coast. Yates and I revel in a beach walk; he is very tolerant that I am unable to walk far, and is particularly fond of the sea and likes to find the pebbles that I throw; he thinks he can jump over the waves, which is fun to watch.

I am a great believer in the saying that 'friends are the family you choose yourself' and I am fortunate to have a very large family, as is evident by the number of Christmas cards I receive and send. Contacts from school, and King's, (we still have reunions at regular intervals) and yet more from Liverpool, Birmingham, and Salisbury and through Dogs for the Disabled are all remembered. Local friends, too many to name, also help with shopping and transport to the hospital, the swimming pool and outings. My general practitioner, and the doctors at Salisbury District Hospital, are very kind and caring, looking after my many helath needs. Despite physical limitations, with the help of my extended family, life is certainly full, for which I count myself fortunate and I want to thank them all. With their help I'll continue walking on wheels.

※ Epilogue ※

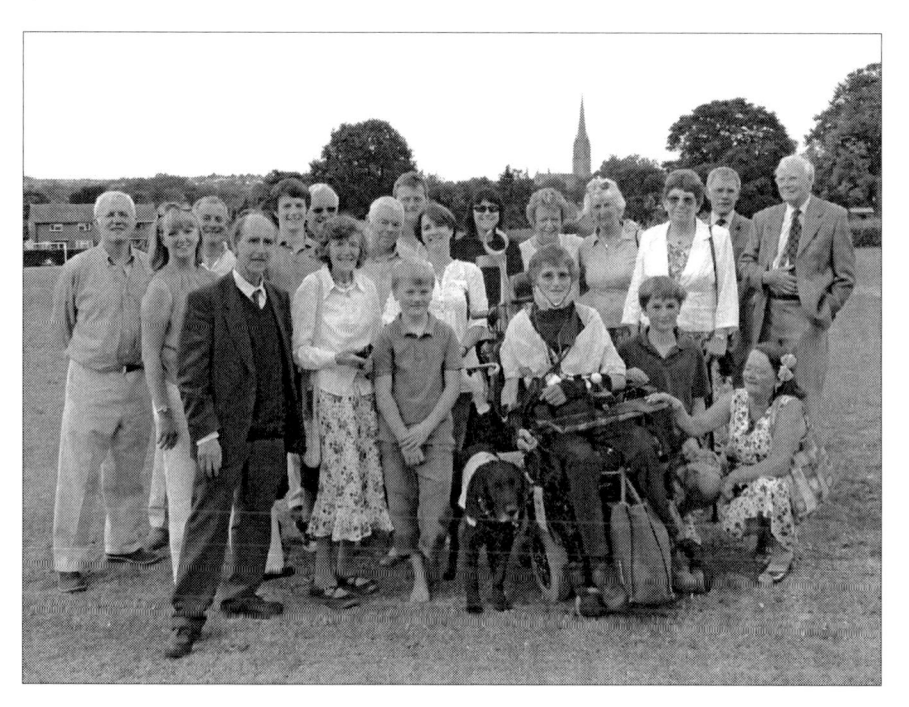

My family and a few of my many friends, June 2011 (photo Michael Camps)

Index

Abbots Bromley, Staffs 92
Acock, Barbara, Derek and family 120, 136, 151
Albert (cat) 89
Alcester, Warwicks 137
Alford, Derek 172
Allan, Martin and Doffy 157, 158
Allerton, Maggie 157
Anderson, Archdeacon 3, 5
Anderson, Dr John 58, 61, 147
Anderson, Professor 125, 127, 129-30, 133, 153, 159-61
Anne, Princess (Princess Royal) 119, 168
Arctic, Bishop of 75
Astrid (dog) 176-80, 183
Atholl House 54, 56, 57, 64
Australia 83, 107, 116

Barford St Martin, Wilts 183
Barnack, Northants 63, 134
Barrett, Jenny 168, 183
Basingstoke, Hants 19
Bates, Harry 144
Battle, Sussex 19
Beavis, Wendy 126-7, 129, 137, 139, 142, 149-51, 156
Beddow, Mr 101, 123
Belgrave Children's Hospital 36
Birmingham 15, 104, 108-61 (passim), 184
    Bishop's Croft 108-9, 111-14, 121, 137-9, 147, 149

Canon Hill 146, 148
Cathedral 120-1
Children's Hospital 109, 112, 114-16, 124, 126, 131
Festival Chorus 120, 141
Four Oaks 137
General Hospital 124, 126, 135
Grove Park 118
Harborne 109, 112, 117-18, 139, 146
Ladywood 118, 147
Oratory 121-2
Queen Elizabeth Hospital 116, 118, 120, 125, 142, 143, 146-8
Selly Oak 130
Winson Green Prison 118
Yardley Wood 138
Bishop, Dr 41, 42
Blackheath 1, 3, 4, 6-8, 13, 14, 19, 24, 31, 33, 35, 43, 50, 52, 57, 122-3, 150, 153
    High School 10-11
Blanch, Bishop Stuart 90
Blundellsands, Merseyside 108
Bootle, Merseyside 63
Blythburgh, Suffolk 122
Boyd, Gillian 17, 18, 28, 34, 43, 53
Boyd, Margaret 89
Brands Hatch 49, 69
Branscombe, Devon 86, 137
Branson, Richard 168
Brennan, Mr 143
Bridges, Miss 72, 73, 76

Index

British Driving Society 168
BROWN, Jill
- aunts and uncles 19-20, 22-3, 29, 34-5, 37, 43, 45, 47, 65-8, 72-3, 86, 89, 91, 95, 96, 100, 108, 111, 135-6, 138-9, 149
- boyfriends 27, 46, 49, 54, 88, 107
- car maintenance 74, 89
- carriage driving 165-8
- cars 70, 91, 110, 121, 130, 135, 145
- childhood 1-25
- church attendance 34-5, 42
- cousins 65, 89
- cycling 9, 66, 87
- death of parents and sister 174-5
- diagnosis 153-61
- dressmaking 68, 100, 108
- driving lessons and tests 47, 56, 60, 62, 65, 66, 69
- grandparents 6, 22
- health problems 24-5, 36, 41, 49, 53, 58-9, 65, 68, 71, 97-110, 123-30, 142-7, 153-61
- holidays 19-24, 30, 47-8, 69, 91-7, 102, 104-6, 122-3, 133-5, 149-52, 183-4
- metalwork 90-1, 100
- move to Salisbury 162
- music 107, 120, 137, 139-41, 147-8, 150, 154-5, 174
- parents, passim
- physiotherapy exams 33, 44-6, 53, 59
- physiotherapy training 18, 28, 31-7, 41-3, 45-7, 48-51, 52-9
- pottery making 67, 146
- registered disabled 143
- rehabilitation 143-4
- riding 164-5
- schools 4, 10-12, 18
- sisters, Elisabeth and Petrena, passim
- sports 12, 28, 42-4, 52, 62, 65-6, 74, 86-8, 98-100
- swimming 126, 129, 136, 141, 148, 170-1
- teaching 116
- woodwork 89-90, 155
- work as physiotherapist 62-3, 67, 72-7, 78-99, 100-4, 114-16, 123-5, 127, 130-3
- writing 85, 101, 104, 116, 160, 169-70, 174

Brown, Vera 157
Brownsea Island, Dorset 135
Bull, Frank 54
Burgess, Pat 164
Burne-Jones, Edward 121
burns (trauma) 82
Burns, Robert 66
Buxton, Ada 156

Cambridge 19, 46, 47, 69, 92
Camps, Michael 138-9, and passim (JB's brother-in-law)
Canada 149
Caney, Doreen 125, 142, 144
Carden, Miss 58
cardio-thoracic disease 114-15
Carriage Driving for the Disabled 160, 165, 167-8
Carrick, Biddy 49, 137, 156, 183
cerebral palsy 80-4, 101, 103-4, 115-16
Chapman, Dorothy 145
Charlton, London 4
Cheshire Homes 54, 173
Chester 63, 73
Chetwynd, Sir Arthur 148-9, 155
Chislehurst, Kent 9
Christmas 8, 39, 60-1, 67, 90, 91, 120, 136-7
Clark, Ernie 61
Clatterbridge Hospital, Wirral 67
Claydon, Dr 53, 58
Cornwall 142
Coventry 141

Cowsill, Mrs 141, 147
Critchley, Freda 108, 136, 156
Cropper, Annie 39, 62
Crosbie, Annette 180
Croydon 151
Crystal Palace, London 136
Cuddesdon, Oxon 35
cystic fibrosis 115

Davies, Ann, Barry and family 63, 134
Davies, Gordon 52
Davies, Mr and Mrs 153, 156
Dee (Lisle), Pat 34, 69, 122, 129, 133
Deganwy, Wales 70
De Garis, Sue 174
Denmark Hill, London 31, 50, 52
Dennis, Carole 63
Derham, Dr 80
Dickens, Iris 121, 138
dogs
    Andy 3, 14, 15, 38
    Astrid 176-80, 183
    Ben 3, 14
    Judy 15, 39, 43-4, 88, 89, 110, 129, 136
    Suki 16, 96, 129, 149
    Yates 170, 171, 174, 180-5
Donhead, Wilts
    Swan Lake Cottage, Higher Coombe 69, 70, 92-7, 104-5, 135, 139, 149
Dorchester 35, 95, 135, 138, 139
Dragonetti, Tricia 174
Downs syndrome 83
Droitwich, Worcs 138
Dulwich, London 54, 157, 158
Dumfries, Scotland 66
    Crichton Royal Hospital 66
Dunwich, Suffolk 122
Durham 73
Dwyer, Mr 98
Dykes, Dr Peter 126, 127, 130, 142, 143

Eastbourne, Sussex 23
Easton, Suffolk 23
Edinburgh 134
    Duke of 119
Elizabeth II, Queen 119
Elphick, Muriel 156
Eltham, London 28, 29, 34, 35, 48, 53
Epping Forest, Essex 13
Evans, Eric 114

Forfar, Scotland 47
Formby, Merseyside 39, 67-8, 89, 91, 151
Foster, Dr 145
Friern Barnet, London 156
Fry, Louise 165

Glamis Castle, Scotland 48
Glen Ceriog, Scotland 48
Gloucester 104, 151
Grasmere, Cumbria 22-3, 96-7, 139
Green, Canon 3
Green, Bishop Mark 150
Green (Murphy), Prudence 18, 69
Greenwich, London 14, 17, 34, 133, 150, 151, 153
Guides, Girl 4, 13, 63-4, 70, 74, 75, 86, 90
Guildford, Surrey 43
Guillain Barré syndrome 84, 104
Gwyn, Sandra 88, 89

Hampson, Bob and Sue 57, 156
Hanning, Caragh, Hugh and James 17, 119, 123, 153
Harefield Hospital, Middlesex 54
Harrison, Mr 143, 146
Hartland, Devon 23
Hathaway, Karen and family 132-3
Hawkins, Dr Clifford 124
Hawkshead, Cumbria 96
Hazlehurst, Mrs 137, 141
Hearn, Dr George 147, 156

* Index *

Heath, Edward 120
Heaton, Ilsa and Joe 148
Henkel, Martin, Mary and family 8, 44, 48, 52, 123
Henley in Arden, Warwicks, 118
Herne Hill, London 31, 54-5, 57, 133, 158, 173
Heveningham Hall, Suffolk 14
Hildrew, Jenny and Robin 135, 139
Hodges, Dudley and Marjorie 35
Hollis, Tessa 156
Honey, Dr G E 65, 98, 100
Horsham, Sussex 22
Houghton, 'Reggie' 5, 52
Hudson, Dr 145
Hughes, Bronwen 79
Hughes, Dr John 79
Huntingfield, Suffolk 14, 20-1
Hunton, Shirley and family 87, 108

International Year for Disabled People 172-3

Jefferies, Jacqueline 151, 154
Jenkinson, Margaret 54, 57, 133, 136, 141, 156
Jobson, Miss 42
Judy (dog) 15, 39, 43-4, 88, 89, 110, 129, 136

Kabity, Doris and Hazel 39, 117-18, 123, 134, 136, 139, 148, 151
Kennington, London 35
Kenya 138
Keswick, Cumbria 66
Kidbrooke, London 1, 4, 37
Kidderminster, Worcs 125
King, Christine 146
Kircudbright, Scotland 66
Knill, Herefs 152

Lambden, Daphne and David 184
Lambert, Angela, Tony and family 85-7, 137-8
Lee, Jenny 142
Leigh-Smith, Miss 56, 65
Lewis, Margaret, 183-4
Lewisham, London 29, 31
  Greyladies 51, 52, 53
Lichfield, Staffs 35, 137
Lill, John 137
Liverpool 12, 15, 34, 35, 38-41, 43-5, 47-8, 53, 55-6, 60-1, 63, 65, 151, 184
  Alder Hey Hospital 50, 75-104 (passim), 107
  Broadgreen General Hospital 85, 98, 100
  Cathedral 37, 60-1, 71, 90, 91, 134
  City Council 72
  Crosby (Great Crosby) 15, 39, 71, 77, 85-7, 91, 137, 144
  Croxteth 38
  Cupplesfield 71, 77, 87, 88-9, 107
  Greenbank School 72-7
  Myrtle Street Hospital 77, 80, 85
  Parkhouse Nursing Home 75, 103
  Playhouse 40
  Royal Liverpool Hospital 100
  Sandfield Park 15, 38, 71-2
  Sandfield Park Special School 116
  Sefton Park 73
  Walton General Hospital 56, 59, 62-3, 72, 85, 91
  West Derby 35, 38-9, 61, 63, 64, 86
  Whiston Hospital 101, 123
London 1, 2, 4, 26-7, 41, 57; and see places separately indexed
  Buckingham Palace 118-19, 138, 155
  Guys Hospital 25, 27, 34, 37, 136
  House of Lords 141
  Kings College Hospital 17, 25, 31-7, 123, 127-9, 133, 136, 147, 153-61, 184
  Mansion House 54

- 189 -

Rodney Street 65
St Bartholomews Hospital 29, 69
Longford Castle and Park, Wilts 165-7, 169
Luton, Beds 1, 6, 19, 49, 122, 137

MacLaren, Morna 165, 168
McPhail, Mrs 7, 49
Maguire, Jean 79
Majorca 102, 105-6, 123
Malawi 136
Margaret, Princess 149
Marshall, Becky, Lizzie and William 6
Martin, Bishop Clifford 34, 40, 90
Menuhin, Yehudi 137
Millar, Anthony 147
Miller, Dr 25
Minsmere, Suffolk 122
Mitchell, Annie 49, 55
Morgan, Dr David 127, 143
Morris, Ethel and Frank 105, 123
Morton, Miss 10
Murphy, Hazel 116
Muscular Dystrophy Group 173-4

National Provident Institution 18, 26-8, 41
Nepean, Susan 42
Newcastle upon Tyne 144-5
North Harrow, London 55
Norton, Stockton on Tees 37, 43, 56, 69, 72, 75-6, 88, 111
Nunton and Bodenham, Wilts 29, 163

Odstock, Wilts 29, 163
Old Radnor, Wales 152
Ormskirk, Lancs 108
Orpington, London 122, 128, 133, 151, 156
Osbourne, Mr 100-1

paralysis 84
Parkes, Prof David 159

Parsons, Dorothy 18
Patrick, Miss 126
Patterson, Sheila 151
Pearce, Dr Alan 111, 123, 147
Pearson, Mr 124, 127
Pembrokeshire, Wales 150
Peterborough, Cambs 134
Petersfield, Hants 173
Philp, Sue 116
Pichler, Gladys 69, 122, 128-9, 133, 151, 156
Pichler, Mary, Peter and family 7-8, 23, 29, 37, 43, 44, 48, 49, 52, 129
Pollock, John 89
Pont Fadog, Wales 134
Poole, Dorset 135
Poppleton, Libby 174
Possum machine 141
Pracey, Mr 98, 101

REMAP 170-1, 174, 180
Reindorp, Bishop George 29, 43, 163
Richard, Cliff 119
Riding for the Disabled Association 160, 164, 169
Robinson, Bishop John, and Ruth 35, 37, 42-4, 47, 50
Rockcliffe, Scotland 66
Roe, John 168
Roehampton Hospital, London 56
Rogers, James and Joyce 66, 134
Rome, Italy 150
Ross, Dorothy 79
Ross, Dr Jimmy, Frances and Evan 25
Royal National Institute for the Blind 146
Royston, Herts 69
Rubin, Mr 75, 77, 80, 86, 103

St Albans, Herts 111, 122, 128, 137, 156
Salisbury 27, 35, 69, 80, 91, 93, 96, 104, 120, 121, 137, 148, 149, 152, 157, 162-85

Index

Cathedral 170, 180, 182
Harnham Bridge 162-3
Post Office 172
St Johns Chapel 157, 162-3
St Johns Singers 174
St Nicholas Hospital 157, 162-3
Sands, Olive 50, 52, 57
Sausman, Alvon 63, 85
Scott, Pauline 82
Scott, Peter 13-14
Scouts, Boy 13, 135
Sedbergh 135
Shaftesbury, Dorset 69, 92, 95, 104
Shotton, Margaret 152
Shrewton, Wilts 152
Simpson, Bishop Bertram, and Joan 5, 57
Small, Dr Michael 142
Smith, Ann Hardy 87
Smith, Joy Whiting 156
Snowdon, Lord 173
Solihull, W Midlands 136
Solva, Wales 55-6
South London Church Fund 1, 3, 29, 61
Southampton General Hospital 180
Southgate, Miss 54
Southport, Merseyside 79
Southwark Catherdal and diocese 4-5, 28, 29, 36, 37, 43, 121, 151, 163
Southwold, Suffolk 14, 22
spina bifida 81-2, 115
Stafford 35
Stamford, Lincs 134
Standish, Lancs 70
Statham, Margaret and John 91, 96
Stewart, Catherine 103
Stewart, Dorothy 72, 74-5, 86, 103, 110, 123, 134, 151
Stewart, Edna 75
Stewart, Evelyn 32, 45, 53, 56, 59, 61
Stiffkey, Norfolk 24
Stoke Mandeville, Bucks 56
Stratford Tony, Wilts 165

Stratford upon Avon, Warwicks 137
Stratton, near Bude, Cornwall 137, 156, 183
Stroud, Tony, Madeline and family 69, 92-7, 104, 136, 149, 157
Stockton on Tees, see Norton
Sweden 18, 23
Sydenham, London 34
Sydling St Nicholas, Dorset 35

Thompson, Georgina 148
Thompson, Jean 63, 72
Thurlow Park, London 36, 48, 53
Tilley, Miss 142
Todd, Dr Robert 79
Toronto, Canada 149
Trickett, Stanley 152
Turland, Alfred 111-12, 116, 117, 119

United States 168-9
  Boston 168
  Maryland 168-9
  Washington 168-9
Uttoxeter, Staffs 92

Walberswick, Suffolk 21-2, 122
Walkden, Mr 99
Walton, Professor 144, 145
Ward-Lilley, Brian 28, 29 and passim (JB's brother-in-law)
Warrington, Cheshire 34
Webster, Dr 101
Welch, Pamela 57
Welwyn Garden City, Herts 1, 2, 3, 24, 122, 133
Wenhaston, Suffolk 30
West Bromwich, West Midlands 112, 118
West Grimstead, Wilts 168
Westerham, Kent 13
Weston, Stuart and Kathleen and family 16, 122, 156
Whipsnade Zoo 136

Whistler, Benedicta 19, 49, 150, 151, 156
White, Pat 34
Whitehouse, Sheila 120
Wibaut, Frank 141, 146, 151
Williamson, Joy 147
Wilson, Bishop Leonard 110
Wilson, Susan 14, 129, 156
Wilton, Wilton House, Wilts 164
Win Green, Wilts 104
Windsor Castle, Berks 14

Wirral, Cheshire 63
Wolfe, Ruth 144
Woolton, Merseyside 40
Woolwich Polytechnic, London 12, 18, 28
Wythall Animal Sanctuary 16

Yates (dog) 170, 171, 174, 180-5
York 67
    Archbishop of 90
    Minster 35, 36

Walking on Wheels